PDQ
MEDICAL GENETICS

RONALD G. DAVIDSON, MD
Consultant Geneticist,
Hospital for Sick Children,
Toronto

Professor Emeritus, Departments of Pediatrics
and Pathology, McMaster University

with illustrations by
Monique Guilderson, BSc, MSc.BMC

2002

BC Decker Inc

Hamilton • London

BC Decker Inc
20 Hughson Street South
P.O. Box 620, L.C.D. 1
Hamilton, Ontario L8N 3K7
Tel: 905-522-7017; 1-800-568-7281
Fax: 905-522-7839; 1-888-311-4987
e-mail: info@bcdecker.com
website: www.bcdecker.com

02 03 04 / CP/ 9 8 7 6 5 4 3 2 1

ISBN 1-55009-178-6

Printed in Canada

Sales and Distribution

United States
BC Decker Inc
P.O. Box 785
Lewiston, NY 14092-0785
Tel: 905-522-7017; 1-800-568-7281
Fax: 905-522-7839; 1-888-311-4987
e-mail: info@bcdecker.com
website: www.bcdecker.com

Canada
BC Decker Inc
20 Hughson Street South
P.O. Box 620, L.C.D. 1
Hamilton, Ontario L8N 3K7
Tel: 905-522-7017; 1-800-568-7281
Fax: 905-522-7839; 1-888-311-4987
e-mail: info@bcdecker.com
website: www.bcdecker.com

Japan
Igaku-Shoin Ltd.
Foreign Publications Department
3-24-17 Hongo, Bunkyo-ku
Tokyo 113-8719, Japan
Tel: 81 3 3817 5680
Fax: 81 3 3815 6776
e-mail: fd@igaku-shoin.co.jp

U.K., Europe, Scandinavia, Middle East
Elsevier Science
Customer Service Department
Foots Cray High Street
Sidcup, Kent   DA14 5HP, UK
Tel: 44 (0) 208 308 5760
Fax: 44 (0) 181 308 5702
e-mail: cservice@harcourt_brace.com

Singapore, Malaysia, Thailand,
Philippines, Indonesia, Vietnam, Pacific
Rim, Korea
Elsevier Science Asia
583 Orchard Road
#09/01, Forum
Singapore 238884
Tel: 65-737-3593
Fax: 65-753-2145

Australia, New Zealand
Elsevier Science Australia
Customer Service Department
STM Division
Locked Bag 16
St. Peters, New South Wales, 2044
Australia
Tel: 61 02 9517-8999
Fax: 61 02 9517-2249
e-mail: stmp@harcourt.com.au
website: www.harcourt.com.au

Foreign Rights
John Scott & Company
International Publishers' Agency
P.O. Box 878
Kimberton, PA 19442
Tel: 610-827-1640
Fax: 610-827-1671
e-mail: jsco@voicenet.com

Notice: The authors and publisher have made every effort to ensure that the patient care recommended herein, including choice of drugs and drug dosages, is in accord with the accepted standard and practice at the time of publication. However, since research and regulation constantly change clinical standards, the reader is urged to check the product information sheet included in the package of each drug, which includes recommended doses, warnings, and contraindications. This is particularly important with new or infrequently used drugs.

To my parents, Lil and Lou Davidson

Acknowledgments

- *To my wife, Miriam, without whose encouragement and school teacher's eye this book would not have been even readable, never mind literate.*

- *Staying within the family, to my son, Alan PhD, Department of Molecular and Medical Genetics and Biochemistry, University of Toronto, Canada, for keeping me au courant with molecular developments; and to my son, Rob commercial photographer, for his help with some of the photos but more important, for guiding his technologically-impaired father out of one computer catastrophe after another during the writing of the manuscript and its submissions to the publisher.*

- *To Barton Childs, Johns Hopkins University and Hospital, my mentor and friend, whom I hope will forgive me if I've inadvertently used his words and phrases, so many of which I've adopted as my own over the years.*

- *To Harry Harris, the father of modern Human Biochemical Genetics, about whom I would say the same as for Barton Childs—mentor and friend, and who was truly the most unforgettable character I've ever had the pleasure of knowing.*

- *To Margaret MacGillivray and Lynn Godmilow, colleagues and friends who contributed their expertise and criticisms to selected chapters, and to Sheila Unger, my former student and now my teacher (the happiest metamorphosis!), who critically appraised the chapter on bone dysplasias.*

- *To Faith Hickman-Brynie and Manert Kennedy, educators par excellence, from whom I learned so much about the basics of teaching and learning, and who got me started on this book during a sabbatical year.*

- *And finally, to all the students, residents and fellows I've taught over the years and from whom I have learned so very much.*

Thank you, thank you, thank you.

Preface

The world does not need yet another standard text on genetics for medical students or any other students for that matter. And what is a "standard text"? Most contain chapters on chromosomes, mitosis and meiosis, biochemical and molecular genetics, mendelian patterns of inheritance, multifactorial disorders, and so on. Several are excellent and will serve the student needing to learn the basics well.[1-3]

So why this book? In addition to meeting an obvious need for a genetics contribution to the PDQ series, what I've attempted to do is present an approach to solving clinical problems. I have made no attempt to cover all problems with issues relevant to genetics, but I hope that the relatively few that have been selected will provide the necessary background and guidelines applicable to most, if not all. In addition, in chapter 1 I've included a few topics that tend not to be covered in the standard texts, along with what I hope will be some helpful hints that I've picked up over the years.

Because this is a problem-based book featuring approaches and with an emphasis on how to find further information on your own through Web sites, patient and family support groups, current literature, and indeed, other books, perhaps the half-life of the text will be increased. Facts go out of date rapidly; approaches require only modification as new advances emerge. In addition, the sheer volume of both old and new information in biology and medicine underlines the need for a conceptual framework within which to sort it all out. Furthermore, mechanisms must be designed to involve students in the personal and social implications and to help them understand the nature of genetics and how its principles flow from those of evolution and natural selection. As stated so appropriately by Barton Childs, "The most enlightened…educators ask not 'What should the student know?' but 'How can we best prepare their minds for what, in time, they will come to know?'"[3]

With the exception of chapter 1, "Introduction to Human Genetics", each chapter in this book begins with a clinical scenario, and the emphasis is on solving the problem presented. Is it then merely a clinically oriented exposition more or less devoid of basic principles? Certainly not! The aim is to have the student recognize the applications of basic science data learned previously in courses and through experience before or during medical school or acquired through grappling with the issues raised in these problems. In addition, the student will be directed to deal with solving the patient's or family's personal difficulties as raised by the scenarios. Each of the clinical scenarios represents either problems requiring knowledge of genetics with which the practicing physician will have to come to grips fairly frequently, or problems that illustrate important basic principles using clinical examples that are not so common. Regarding the latter, I tried to use topics that in general have not been very clearly approached in most of the standard texts recommended for medical students. I think it is safe to say that the general approaches outlined in this text will not change so very much over the ensuing years, although clearly the specific details will, including, especially, new diagnostic and treatment modalities. Thus, I have tried to avoid inclusion of detailed descriptions of either the basic science or the clinical aspects, emphasizing instead how to go about obtaining the latest molecular testing information, the latest imaging techniques, and so on that might help solve the problems. One of my favorite old Chinese proverbs is, "Give me a fish and I will eat for a day. Teach me how to fish and I will eat for a lifetime."

In the "old days" of medical genetics, we dealt with rare diseases, almost all of which were monogenic (mendelian); they were of great interest to the affected individuals and their families, and were managed for the large part by geneticists. Most of even the current textbooks devote the bulk of their pages to the mendelian disorders and chromosomal aberrations.

The **new genetics** is very different; nine out of 10 of the leading causes of mortality have genetic components, and the one that is usually considered not to, accidents[4], might also be included if you believe that there are genetic components to risk-taking behaviors and other activities that predispose to being a victim of trauma. Care is being provided increasingly by family physicians and specialists other than geneticists.

Obviously, there is a need for physicians to learn to think genetically—to recognize genetic factors and to learn to explain genetics to patients. In addition, and perhaps most importantly, society needs to prepare for the new genetics. We as medical people must participate in the implementation of the learning of principles of genetics in schools and in the training of business people who will have to deal with insurance companies, issues of privacy regarding genetic testing of employees, and with the need to share in the funding of basic as well as applied research, so that the exciting advances already made will continue.

I find it curious that even as we are well into the molecular age, texts in human genetics continue to begin with chapters on chromosomes, mendelian segregation of diseases, and pedigrees. Does it not make sense to begin with the gene, from which all the rest of our subject derives?! So let us remedy that for this book.

What Is a Gene?

The student of today will immediately provide a practical definition probably more or less as follows: a gene is a section of a strand of deoxyribonucleic acid (DNA) that is responsible for encoding an amino acid chain that will, either on its own or in combination with other identical or nonidentical amino acid chains, make proteins; some proteins will function as enzymes and others as components of the structure of organs and tissues. Many students will add that some sections of the DNA act as regulatory elements. The base pairs that make up the genetic material, the various ribonucleic acids (RNAs), and the assembly of proteins on the ribosomes presumably will be described. The well-informed student might add that the order of the base pairs in the strand is susceptible to change by mutation and crossing over, and that the strand itself represents the basic unit of recombination.

That's not bad for a start but the true, almost awesome *wonder* of the genetic material is being missed. Let us consider, briefly, some of these wonders, which emerge from a broader look at the definition and function of the gene. Often a historical examination, even as brief a one as the following, can be beneficial.

Long before Mendel, observant physicians noted the familial nature of some types of human illness, anticipating the concept that genes, when changed or mutated, can be responsible for a disease or a predisposition to a disease. And it wasn't just physicians who made these seminal observations. The Talmud, the ancient collection of Jewish law and tradition, notes that male siblings of infants who bleed excessively at circumcision should not themselves be circumcised, and on the basis of further observation and deduction, they proscribed the ritual for male cousins on the maternal side of the family, recognizing the pattern of X-linked inheritance if not the mechanism.

Gregor Mendel, born in 1822, recognized the existence of hereditary factors that *segregate* (they are transferred unchanged from one generation to the next) and *assort* independently. As the saying goes, it is better to be lucky than clever, but Mendel was both! Luck came with his choice of phenotypes to test; the traits were discontinuous (e.g., tall versus short plants, wrinkled versus smooth seed surfaces), there was no lack of penetrance, and the traits were not genetically linked (linked loci are on the same chromosome). His aim was to learn about probability and the role of hybridization.

Charles Darwin, born in 1809, pondered the issues of evolution through studies of normal variation in plants and animals resulting primarily from natural selection. In spite of their being contemporaries, they never met and Darwin knew nothing about Mendel's **hereditary factors**. Yet Darwin's concept, put in relatively modern terms, can be stated thus: the living organism undergoes random mutations that, in a sense, it presents to its own unique environment. That environment then disposes of these variants in a variety of ways—those that present some sort of advantage will be preserved and provide some improvement of the species, while others might contribute to the generation of a new species. The harmful ones will be eliminated either through lethality or decreased fitness.

Francis Galton, Darwin's first cousin, studied humans, eschewing variation in order to examine how relatives *resemble* each other; that is, he looked at traits such as height and intelligence for correlations and showed how such continuous traits regressed toward the mean (e.g., extremely intelligent parents' offspring tend on the average to be less intelligent than their progenitors). R.A.Fisher, the British mathematician, concluded correctly that both discontinuous and continuous variation are a consequence of mendelian genes.

Griffith uncovered the **transforming principle** of the bacterium pneumococcus as a bacterial extract that could change the configuration of the capsule. Then Avery, McLeod, and MacCarty demonstrated that the transforming principle was DNA and that the genetic information was carried only in the DNA.

Yanofsky demonstrated the colinearity of sequences of base pairs with sequences of amino acids in proteins, and the X-ray crystallographers laid the groundwork for the model, the double helical structure, that was sorted out by Watson and Crick.

Beadle and Tatum proposed that genes specified proteins, one gene for one protein, but problems with the structural concept emerged almost immediately. Monod and Jacob found that in *Escherichia coli* part of the DNA appeared to regulate two structural genes. The so-called **operator** could undergo mutation but made no protein product. Later, the existence of regulatory sequences located at a distance from the structural gene(s) was discovered. Unfortunately, not much was made of the difference between the genes and the traits that they either specified or to which they contributed, which is a problem that continues to blur some of our thinking even today.

Things got more complicated when it was discovered that the molecules of nuclear RNA were much larger than cytoplasmic messenger RNA (mRNA), which led to the discovery of introns and exons, the former being spliced out of the nuclear mRNA.

And have you started to feel a bit queasy as data from the Human Genome Project are indicating that the number of genes will turn out to be closer to 35,000 rather than the earlier estimates of 80,000 to 100,000? How can so few genes encode the blueprint for an organism as complex as a human being? Part of the answer lies in the discovery that although DNA is usually transcribed in only one direction, occasionally a transcript is made from the other strand. The base-pair sequence is read in the opposite direction and thus specifies an entirely different protein. Both molecules are genes but they come from just one sequence of base pairs. Furthermore, one transcript could contain the information to encode two or more proteins— is that transcript one gene or two? Similarly, one transcript can produce an enzyme with multiple active sites with several activities.

It gets even more intriguing. One RNA transcript can be processed in such a way as to produce two or more different proteins through alternative splicing. And the human genome is anything but static; we have DNA sequences that migrate (jumping genes or transposons) and trinucleotide repeats of highly variable numbers within the transcribed portion of genes.

Much of the DNA is noncoding and untranscribed; we still don't know what it's doing. Some are partially duplicated gene sequences or pseudo-genes; much is said to be "evolutionary baggage," genes that functioned in ancient ancestors but that serve no purpose in humans and have for some reason remained part of the genome. But who knows?

Advances in molecular aspects continue apace and I will refer to some from time to time throughout the text.

So, after all that, what is a gene?

The practical definition is the molecular structural one: a strand of base pairs in the DNA whose arrangement is reflected in that of the amino acids in the single peptide it specifies. The order and quality of base pairs in the strand is susceptible to change by mutation and crossing over, and the strand itself represents the basic unit of recombination.

The functional definition encompasses different actions in different time frames; for example, self-replication in each mitotic and meiotic cell division, reproduction of individuals, developmental maturation and then aging of individuals over time and throughout the life cycle of the individual, and the specification of the proteins that maintain homeostasis. Thus, the genes' function, other than in reproduction, is strictly to specify the structure of peptides; the business of the cell is transacted without further reference to those genes. Again, beware the tendency to ascribe to the gene capabilities that actually reside in their products.

And finally, to the educator, "the gene represents the options and constraints within which each individual forms the developmental trajectories that prepare him to face adaptively his experiences of the environment."[3]

I cannot close this preface without paying particular tribute to my mentor and friend, the educator Barton Childs. His book[3] is a must read for any serious student of the role of genetics in medicine. Each chapter should be savored in the true sense of that word and revisited. For a more thorough exposition of "what is a gene," read and enjoy chapter 14 at the very least.

Ronald G. Davidson
March 2002

References

1. Nussbaum RL, McInnes RR, Willard HF. Thompson and Thompson genetics in medicine. 6th ed. Toronto: WB Saunders; 2001.
2. Motulsky AG, Vogel F. Human genetics: problems and approaches. 3rd ed. Berlin: Springer Verlag; 1997.
3. Childs B. Genetic medicine. A logic of disease. Baltimore: Johns Hopkins University Press; 1999.
4. Deaths and death rates for the 10 leading causes of death in specified age groups: United States, preliminary 1995 http://www.geocities.com/CapeCanaveral/3504/topten.htm (last accessed February 2002).

Contents

PDQ
Medical Genetics

Introduction to Human Genetics

What students will find in this somewhat unusual introduction are the "few topics" to which I referred in the preface. They are issues that are a bit difficult to work into a problem-based format but that are essential for students to tackle. No attempt will be made to be complete; this is as advertised—an introduction—as well as an attempt to include some observations that I've made over the years that might be helpful. The references and Web sites will provide the details for those who wish to do some additional reviewing.

MENDELIAN GENETICS AND SINGLE-GENE INHERITANCE

Perhaps some of my readers have already concluded, just from the preface, that with rare exceptions, single-gene inheritance really doesn't exist in humans. The path from a mutation in a single gene to a phenotype is rarely straightforward,[1] and many mendelian traits fulfill the criteria for **complex conditions** (see chapter 2, "Complex Genetic Disorders"). Think about eye color, a normal, so-called dominant trait. In all those old textbooks where we "learned" that brown is dominant over blue, why didn't anyone ask where green and hazel and all those other lovely variations in iris color come from? Or take a simple autosomal recessive disease such as phenylketonuria. There are multiple causative mutations and more than one locus involved, and without a fairly high protein intake, there might be no disease at all regardless of which mutation the patient might have (see chapter 5, "Newborn Screening"). However, we are stuck with the terms **dominant** and **recessive** and have to deal with them at a practical level; that is, in patient counseling.

Autosomal Dominant Inheritance

Note that at no time have I used the term **dominant genes**: genes don't dominate anything; they just code for amino acid chains. The polypeptide chains then carry out the business of the cell or mess it up if they are sufficiently abnormal.

Why, since genes come in pairs, would one abnormal member of a pair have any effect at all on the phenotype of the individual possessing it? The other member of that pair, that is, the other allele, ought to be able to make enough product to allow normal function. *Stop* at this point—you should be able to come up with at least three ways for a mutation to have a dominant effect. Don't cheat; write them down before you look at the next section!

OK, here they are:

1. **Totally nonfunctional allele**. Sometimes half a product just isn't enough, as in some cases of osteogenesis imperfecta, fragile bone disease.[2]
2. **Abnormal polypeptide chains**. Sometimes the abnormal polypeptide chains mixed in with normal chains, even in a roughly 50:50 ratio, simply weaken the structure; this is analogous to the chain that is only as strong as its weakest link. Marfan syndrome is a good example. The poor-quality connective tissue of the aortic root cannot handle the tremendous pressure generated by the systolic contractions of the heart over time, and it slowly breaks down with expansion of the root. That can lead to a tear in the epithelial lining, which cannot expand to accommodate the expanded root, hence the dissecting aneurysm, or sometimes to a rupture of the aorta itself with sudden death.
3. **Protein structure**. The structure of the protein involved can be important. In one type of osteogenesis imperfecta, the mutation affects type 1 collagen, a tissue that is composed of two α-1 (I)-chains and one α-2 (I)-chain; that is, it is a trimer. Obviously, a mutation in the α-1 chain affects not 50% but 75% of the molecule. This is referred to as a dominant negative effect.
4. **Gain-of-function mutations**. Yes, I'm afraid so—there are gain-of-function mutations as well! In achondroplasia (see chapter 7, "Bone Dysplasias and Short Stature"), the causative mutation is a fibroblast growth factor receptor (*FGFR3*) gene. The mutations activate the negative growth control exerted by *FGFR3* and that causes constitutive activation of the FGF receptor and a negative regulation of bone growth. The net result: impaired bone growth. In addition, mutations in oncogenes cause typical gain-of-function: mutations allow suppressed cellular growth genes to reactivate.

What kinds of traits or diseases are likely to show dominant inheritance? Variations in structural proteins have been used as examples above, and that makes sense. In contrast, defects of proteins that function as enzymes tend to be inherited as recessive traits, and again, that is logical: if one allele of a pair makes nothing and the other functions normally, the individual ends up with, on average, 50% of normal activity in the heterozygote and generally that is enough for most enzymatically catalyzed processes to function normally.

Heterogeneity

Heterogeneity is almost the rule for dominant conditions. Think about a couple of the relatively common ones, such as neurofibromatosis or Marfan syndrome. Some individuals with neurofibromatosis, for example, have almost nothing to show for it, perhaps a few café-au-lait spots with freckling in the axillae and groin. Others have multiple small subcutaneous tumors or even quite massive deforming neurofibromas with involvement of many other organ systems. A variety of explanations can account for this genetic heterogeneity, including multiple mutant alleles with different effects, as described above, as well as the realization that these are complex molecules, connective tissue being an example, that are coded by many different genes, only one of which is mutated in a given disease. The mutated gene acts in the milieu of all the others; thus, even siblings will have different alleles at those other loci and hence different modifying effects on the disease-causing one. The end result is intra- as well as interfamilial variability.

Pedigree

Nothing could be easier to predict than the pedigree. The affected individual has one mutant and one normal allele; since we pass our genes to our offspring one member of a pair at a time, the risk of an affected parent having an affected child is 50:50. The numbers of affected males and females ought to be equal. A typical pedigree is shown in Figure 1–1.

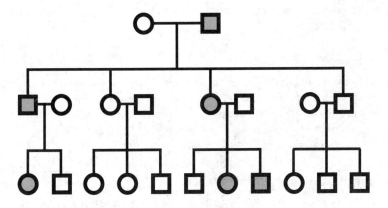

Figure 1–1 Typical autosomal dominant pedigree.

Exceptions are almost the rule rather than the norm. See if you can come up with some of the reasons before reading on.

Here they are:

1. Sex-limited disorders. Although such conditions as male pattern baldness are unquestionably complex disorders, some families show apparent autosomal dominant segregation with lack of expression in females, some of whom do indeed develop postmenopausal partial alopecia.

2. Lack of penetrance (see glossary).

3. Decreased expressivity. Some cases can be so mild as to be entirely missed, especially if the family or the physician is not thoroughly familiar with the total spectrum of the condition, including the very minor manifestations, for example, a single central incisor in familial holoprosencephaly or, as mentioned above, axillary freckling in neurofibromatosis.

4. Germline mutations. The observation to be explained—phenotypically normal parents have not one but two children with, for example, achondroplasia, a typical autosomal dominant condition (see chapter 7, "Bone Dysplasias and Short Stature"). The most likely explanation is a mutation that arose in the developing germline when either the mother or the father was an embryo. Thus, for this relatively rare but well-documented event, one of the parental gonads is populated with an indeterminate number of gametes containing the mutation, and determining the magnitude of the risk for future affected offspring is not possible.

5. Phenocopy. Same observation as above; another possibility—the diagnosis is wrong and whatever the actual form of dwarfism, the cause would be different. The term is used when a condition mimics a well-known phenotype but has a different etiology, usually environmental but not necessarily.

6. False paternity. Same observation again (unlikely in this particular example) but something to keep in mind when pedigrees don't match expectations.

Genetic Counseling

The obvious analogy for genetic counseling is the coin toss, but beware: you really do need to point out that each toss of the coin is an independent event. Sometimes you will toss two, three, four, or even more heads in a row, and no matter how many heads you've tossed, the chance of tossing a head on the next throw is still 50:50.

Autosomal Recessive Inheritance

Figure 1–2 shows a stylized pedigree with the well-known 1-2-1 ratio. Typically, both parents are heterozygous for a mutant allele at the same gene

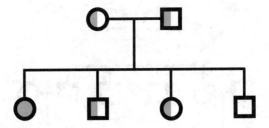

Figure 1–2 Stylized autosomal recessive pedigree.

locus and phenotypically are unaffected by the mutation in a single dose. However, whether or not one considers a carrier as normal depends on how hard one looks and by what means. The carrier of a β-thalassemia mutation, for example, is often mildly anemic, could be mistakenly diagnosed as iron deficient, and might be treated unnecessarily with potentially harmful results due to iron overload. The sickle cell disease carrier is certainly not phenotypically normal if you are looking at his or her blood smear after exposure to a reducing agent. The term **carrier** is a synonym for heterozygote but please do not say "heterozygous carrier"—that is redundant.

The risk of having a homozygous affected offspring is one in four, but beware: people's understanding of odds is often deficient, as exemplified by the almost unbelievable success of casinos and lotteries! Some will conclude that since they have one affected child, the next three children will be unaffected. The deck of cards analogy will usually work. There is a one-in-four chance of drawing a heart, spade, diamond, or club, but there is a game called poker and a hand known as a flush (five cards of the same suit); although fairly rare, it does occur. Obviously, with a one-in-four risk, two or even more affected offspring in a sibship is not so unlikely. If the parents respond that the analogy is faulty because it applies only if you replace each card into the deck and reshuffle before you draw the next one, you will know you have succeeded in making the point!

It is also important to point out that among the unaffected offspring of carrier parents, two out of three will be carriers, on average, and one will be homozygous normal. This seems to be a bit difficult for some to grasp and you need to explain that the affected individual is usually obvious, and that leaves two possibilities for the remaining three hypothetical offspring in the pedigree in Figure 1–2, carrier or homozygous normal, and usually you can't distinguish among them unless there is a biochemical, molecular, or other test. Don't hesitate to draw the typical pedigree for the family you are counseling.

The next pedigree, Figure 1–3, appears to be dominant, but it isn't. It is recessive. Can you think of two possible explanations for what could be called **pseudodominant inheritance**? Easy, right? They are as follows:

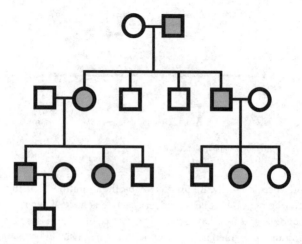

Figure 1–3 Pseudodominant pedigree.

1. Consanguinity (see the shaded portion of Figure 1–4)
2. High prevalence of the mutant allele in the population (the shaded portion in Figure 1–5). Hemochromatosis is a good example. Close to one person in 10 is a carrier in the general population so that even unrelated parents have a fairly high risk of both being carriers ($1/10 \times 1/10$).

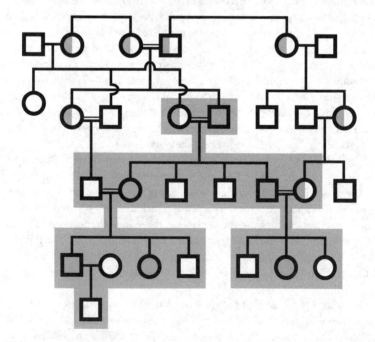

Figure 1–4 Consanguinity to account for pseudodominance.

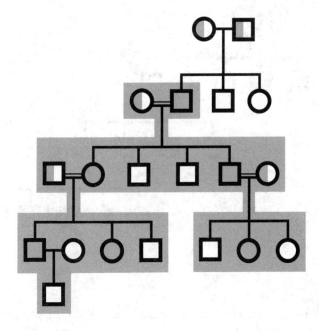

Figure 1–5 High prevalence of the mutant allele to account for pseudodominance.

As with dominant conditions, heterogeneity or variability is the rule, not the exception. Cystic fibrosis is a good example; more than 800 mutant alleles are known and many "homozygous" affected individuals are really compound heterozygotes (they inherited a different mutant allele at the same gene locus from each parent). In addition, modification of expression due to varying alleles at different loci, as well as differing environmental effects, make many recessive conditions more closely resemble complex disorders, as mentioned at the beginning of the chapter.

X-Linked Disorders

Both recessive and dominant X-linked disorders occur, the former being much more common.

X-Linked Recessive Disorders

The pedigree is often described as analogous to the knight's move in chess; a typical example is shown in Figure 1–6. Males are most often affected and receive the gene via their carrier mothers who, typically, are phenotypically

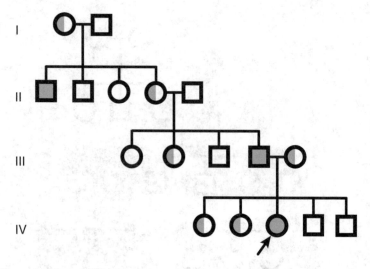

Figure 1–6 Typical X-linked pedigree.

normal. Again, on average, half the sons of a carrier woman will be affected and half the daughters of a carrier woman will be carriers.

Females can be affected on the basis of the following:

- Having a carrier mother and an affected father; i.e., the female marked by the arrow in Figure 1–6 is homozygous for an X-linked mutation.
- Nonrandom X inactivation (see "Exceptions to Mendelian Inheritance," below).

Note:

- Father-to-son transmission of an X-linked trait is impossible; if dad passes his one and only X chromosome to an offspring, the child will be a girl, except under very rare circumstances involving, for example, chromosome translocations.
- Unless we're dealing with a common recessive condition, such as color blindness, the vast majority of affected individuals will be males, in contrast to X-linked dominant conditions (see below).
- Unlike autosomal recessive conditions, consanguinity is irrelevant for X-linked recessive conditions.

X-Linked Dominant Disorders

Since women have twice as many X chromosomes as men, dominant conditions are seen much more frequently among females in the general population. For an affected female, the pedigree appears identical to that of an autosomal dominant one—on average, half the daughters and half the sons will be affected. But for an affected male, things are very different, as shown in Figure 1–7: **all** of the daughters and **none** of the sons are affected. As would be expected, often the manifestations of an X-linked dominant condition in affected males are more severe than in an affected female because of the mitigating influence of the normal allele on the second X. In fact, many X-linked dominant mutations are apparently lethal in males during intrauterine life, further reducing the number of affected males with these diseases. A typical pedigree is shown in Figure 1–8 and demonstrates the following:

- Half the daughters of an affected woman are affected.
- Male embryos that inherit the mutation spontaneously abort.
- None of the liveborn sons is affected (unless, of course, there is a chromosome anomaly, such as Klinefelter's syndrome, 47,XXY).

Note that for many X-linked dominant conditions, most cases are due to new mutations; familial cases are rare.

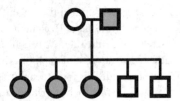

Figure 1–7 X-linked dominant pedigree.

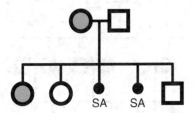

Figure 1–8 X-linked dominant pedigree; mutation lethal in males. SA = spontaneous abortion.

The Y Chromosome

The human Y chromosome is much smaller than the X (about the size of chromosome 22) and has no more than a few dozen genes, as compared to the X chromosome's 2,000 to 3,000. The rest of the chromosome is made up of noncoding sequences of nucleotides, sometimes referred to as junk deoxyribonucleic acid (DNA). Most of the actual Y-linked genes are on the short arm and are allelic with genes on the short arm of the X chromosome. The two sex chromosomes pair at meiosis end to end, obviously very different from the homologous pairing of the autosomes. Among the genes are the so-called housekeeping genes needed for the survival of most cells and a few that participate in male fertility. The *SRY* locus determines male sex and is discussed in chapter 4, "Ambiguous Genitalia". There are no structural genes on the Y and no syndromes or even single physical traits determined by Y-linked genes other than those related to sex determination. Jegalian and Lahn's paper[3] is an easy-to-read description of the "odd couple," the human X and Y chromosomes, concentrating on the Y, including its evolution and role in male infertility.

MITOCHONDRIAL DISORDERS

Figure 1–9 shows a pedigree to conjure with! It's a stylized one for mitochondrial inheritance and shows a unique pattern: only affected females transmit the trait; all the daughters and all the sons of an affected woman are affected, as shown in generations I and II. Generation III is where it gets interesting but this is readily explicable. Again, all the offspring of an affected woman are affected regardless of their sex, but none of the offspring of affected men are affected. This is **maternal inheritance** and results from mitochondrial mutations. Mitochondria in humans are received exclusively from one's mother. Those present in sperm are confined to the tail piece and are shed at fertilization. However, only rarely is such a typical pedigree found for any given family with any given mitochondrial disorder. A variety of factors contributes to the heterogeneity.

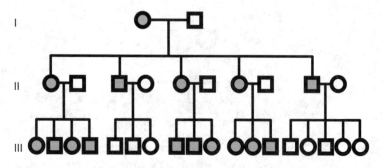

Figure 1–9 Mitochondrial/maternal inheritance: stylized pedigree.

A detailed description of mitochondrial disorders and their heredity is beyond the mission of this book, but some highlights are presented. There are excellent review papers[4,5] and the Web sites for the United Mitochondrial Disease Foundation (click on "For Physician") and the Muscular Dystrophy Association provide very clear and concise information for the neophyte.

What Are Mitochondria?

Mitochondria are the intracellular power plants responsible for the production of high-energy phosphate bonds through activation of adenosine 5′diphosphate (ADP) to adenosine triphosphate (ATP) by oxidative phosphorylation of carbohydrates, fatty acids, or amino acids. Each human cell contains hundreds of mitochondria (with the exception of red blood cells) and thousands of mitochondrial DNAs.

Mitochondrial DNA is double stranded, circular, and 16.5 kilobases long. It codes for 13 polypeptides essential to the enzymes of the mitochondrial energy-generating pathways, plus large and small ribosomal ribonucleic acids (rRNAs) and 22 transfer RNAs (tRNAs) necessary for mitochondrial protein synthesis. It is interesting to note that more than 90% of mitochondrial proteins are coded by *nuclear* DNA—they find their way into the mitochondria from the cytoplasm.

Mitochondrial DNA has a higher mutation rate than nuclear DNA and no enzymatic repair system. The significance of each mutation to human variability and disease depends on where in the genome and when in the human life cycle the mutation occurs. Germ-line mitochondrial DNA mutations can be neutral or deleterious. Neutral and mildly deleterious mutations have accumulated in female lineages for thousands of years; thus, their nature, prevalence, and geographic distribution reflect the prehistory of women, just as Y-linked variations do for men, and they have played a huge role in allowing us to trace radiating female lineages as women migrated from Africa into the various continents during the eons of human evolution.

Mitochondrial DNA has another novel feature: when a mutation first arises within a cell, it creates an intracellular mixture of mutant and normal molecules; this is called **heteroplasmy**. As a heteroplasmic cell divides, it is a matter of chance as to the relative number of mutant and normal DNAs that end up in the daughter cells; the proportion can differ from pure mutant to pure normal mitochondrial populations, a phenomenon known as **homoplasmy**. And we see all variations in between the two homoplasmies. As one would expect, this random distribution of differing populations of mitochondria creates great variability among offspring, even within the same sibship.

Sometimes mutations accumulate in mitochondrial DNAs of *post*mitotic tissues as humans age and they can interfere with normal organ and tissue function. Their potential importance in organ senescence associated with aging and with the diseases of aging, Parkinson's and Alzheimer's disease, for example, is a subject of exciting current research.

Mitochondrial Diseases

As one would expect, organ systems with the highest energy requirements, such as the brain, skeletal muscle, and heart muscle, are most susceptible to damage from mitochondrial mutations. More than 40 mitochondrial disorders have been described in humans, each one quite rare.

Mitochondrial disease should be suspected on the basis of multiple system involvement with unusual combinations of brain or neuromuscular disorders, or both, with or without visual or hearing defects; all manifestations are usually progressive in nature. Typical signs include the following:

- Muscle weakness, myoclonia, loss of muscle control, or incoordination
- Developmental delay
- Visual or hearing impairment

Ages of onset run from before birth to old age. Manifestations are characteristically episodic and often are precipitated by infections or other types of stress (e.g., infection, starvation). A list of mitochondrial diseases can be found on the Web sites listed later, along with descriptions of each, as well as techniques for diagnosis.

Laboratory Testing

Increased likelihood of mitochondrial disease can be determined through fairly simple initial testing that would include the following:

- Blood lactate studies (often elevated)
- Blood sugar studies (diabetes is not uncommon in mitochondrial disorders)
- Metabolic screening, including amino acids, organic acids, ammonia, ketones, fatty acids, and carnitine (a variety of anomalies have been found)

EXCEPTIONS TO MENDELIAN INHERITANCE

I. X Inactivation: The Lyon Hypothesis

Mendel, of course, knew nothing about chromosomes and certainly nothing about sex determination via a heteromorphic sex chromosome pair. The peculiar segregation patterns of genes on the X and Y chromosomes have been discussed, but there's more.

When it was realized that the sex-determining pair of chromosomes in mammals, the X and Y, contained important genes having nothing to do with sex determination (literally thousands of them on the human X chromosome, for example), a puzzle emerged. How could a species tolerate a situation where one sex, the female, had twice as many of these genes as the male and at least the potential for producing twice as much gene product for each of them? Without some compensatory mechanism, one sex would almost certainly have a significant advantage over the other and the disadvantaged sex would, over the eons of evolution, disappear and with it, the entire species!

Mary Lyon, a mouse geneticist, first proposed, on the basis of studies of X-linked coat-color variants, that in the normal mammalian female, one of the two X chromosomes is functionally inactivated. She went on to hypothesize the following:

- The inactivation must occur early in the life of the embryo.
- In each embryonic cell, it is a matter of chance as to which of the two X chromosomes (the paternally or maternally derived one) is inactivated.
- Once an X chromosome is inactivated in an embryonic cell, all the progeny of that cell maintain the same inactive X.
- In individuals with more than two X chromosomes, all those in excess of one are inactivated.

Thus, the normal mammalian female is a mosaic of X chromosome gene expression, with patches of cells expressing the genes of the paternally derived X and patches expressing those of the maternally derived X. On average, the split will be 50:50, but since the inactivation event is random, considerable variation could, and in fact does, occur.

X inactivation is no longer a hypothesis and some very good reviews have been published covering the mechanisms by which the inactivation is brought about, as well as other more recently discovered related phenomena.[6,7] For example, in humans, there are many genes that escape inactivation, whereas in mice, exceptions to inactivation are rare. In addition, X inactivation is not entirely random.

The significance of X inactivation is profound. It was the first example of **genomic imprinting** (see section III below). If you think about it, the act and the consequences of X inactivation are a form of imprinting. Either the paternally or maternally derived X is inactivated and imprinted, since the inactivation is maintained in the progeny of that cell throughout the remaining development and growth of that individual organism.

Clinical Implications of X Inactivation

1. **X-linked recessive disorders**. In many X-linked recessive disorders, the heterozygotes have a remarkable range of expression varying from

being phenotypically normal to manifesting characteristics of the disorder almost as severely, or as severely, as the affected male. In most instances this results from the randomness of X inactivation and the phenomenon is referred to as **skewed inactivation**. However, other factors play roles in this marked variation in expression of X-linked genes and some aspects could be influenced by epigenetic regulation.

2. **X-chromosome aneuploidy**. Males and females with multiple X chromosomes (e.g., in Klinefelter's syndrome, 47,XXY and the triple-X female, 47,XXX) are often phenotypically normal or have relatively minor anomalies, in sharp contrast to autosomal aneuploidy, where almost invariably devastating effects occur, even when there is only partial aneuploidy, as often is the case with tiny unbalanced translocations. Obviously, inactivation of all X chromosomes in excess of one accounts, in large part, for this phenomenon. However, as the number of additional X chromosomes increases, the phenotypical anomalies become progressively more severe. There is little doubt that some of the genes that escape inactivation play a role in the abnormal features of the phenotypes of individuals with X-chromosome aneuploidy.

3. **Immunological phenomena**. Females, on average, have two- to threefold higher incidences of autoimmune diseases, including rheumatoid arthritis, systemic lupus erythematosus, and so on. Although not a direct result of X inactivation, this sex difference is fascinating and probably related, at least in part, to genes on the X chromosome, whether or not they are inactivated. Here is the theory. The structural genes for the immunoglobulins are clearly autosomal, but there are genes responsible for the control of those autosomal genes on the X chromosome. Whatever these controlling genes turn out to be, and however they might function, females have twice as many of them as males and therefore, theoretically, twice the chance of having mutations that could predispose to or actually cause autoimmune disease.

   Along the same line, in the face of infection, immunoglobulins obviously play a major role in our defense mechanisms; thus, females ought to have an advantage over males, whether or not the γ-globulin locus or loci are inactivated. Again, with two X chromosomes as compared with the male's one, the female has the capacity for greater variability in response, at least in relation to whatever genes are on the X. The greater the potential variability in response, the more efficient will be that response. There are data to support this, especially relating to the newborn period,[8] where males and females are as equal from a homeostatic viewpoint as they will ever be (for example, there is at that time relatively little in the way of hormonal differences and relatively little environmental influence). There is a significantly higher infection rate in males.

   Food for thought!

II. Genetic Anticipation

One of the basic concepts established in Mendel's experiments is that genetic factors pass unchanged from generation to generation. Hybridization experiments with, for example, white and red flowers, showed that in the F1 generation there might appear to be blending of parental characteristics (i.e., all the flowers were pink). In the next generation, however, among the progeny of the hybrid cross, the original parental white and red flowers re-emerged—the phenotypes changed but the genes were unaltered.

Then came the observation that in some medical conditions, mostly dominantly inherited neurological or neuromuscular diseases, the age of onset became earlier and the severity of the manifestations worsened as the gene passed from generation to generation.

The phenomenon is known as a **genetic anticipation** and, at least in its early days, its history was nothing of which to be proud.[9] It all began back in the early decades of the 20th century in relation primarily to non-mendelian disorders, notably mental illness. Observations were made of the offspring of mentally handicapped individuals by observers strongly influenced by eugenic concepts of degeneration of the race through unrestricted proliferation of children in families where one or both parents were mentally "dull" or otherwise undesirable. Observers described more severe intellectual deficiencies and earlier onset with successive generations. Such flawed observations as these were among the factors that contributed to the excesses of the Holocaust soon to come.

At about the same time, it was noted in families with myotonic dystrophy, an autosomal dominant disorder, that there were individuals with isolated cataracts (these individuals did not have any detectable muscle disorder) whose descendants showed, in addition to cataracts, muscle weakness and other manifestations of myotonic dystrophy. The first attempt at a detailed study was by Julia Bell in 1947; she clearly showed worsening of clinical signs and earlier onset from generation to generation with statistical analyses to back up those conclusions.

The timing of these studies was bad for at least two reasons. First, there was no discernible explanation for what they were describing, and second, it was just after World War II. One of Bell's colleagues, Lionel Penrose, later to become the Galton professor of human genetics, was an ardent anti-eugenicist and he presented arguments and statistical analyses to show that Bell's observations were biased. Penrose had a profound influence on many aspects of human genetics and Bell's data were ignored. The term **anticipation** disappeared from textbooks and papers in the field until the emergence of a biological basis for it several decades later.

The first indication of the existence of a biological factor causing anticipation in myotonic dystrophy was documented in 1960 with the first clear descriptions of *congenital* myotonic dystrophy. The affected infants were invariably the offspring of affected *mothers*. The nature of the biological factor responsible for this phenomenon was, of course, unknown at the time but the possibility of some maternal metabolite that might cross the placenta during intrauterine development was raised as a possibility.

The next events were very detailed family studies of myotonic dystrophy in the mid-1980s, eventually refuting Penrose's explanation of anticipation as entirely a statistical bias. The studies showed clear and unequivocal intergenerational differences, regardless of the sex of the parent. In 1989, similar family studies done for fragile-X syndrome also showed similarly remarkable intragenerational differences. In 1991, unstable DNA sequences were demonstrated in families with fragile-X syndrome and the underlying molecular phenomenon consisted of variable-length CCG repeat sequences. By the end of that year, unstable DNA sequences in myotonic dystrophy were also demonstrated and were confirmed by additional studies in 1992.

Now there are more than a dozen neurodegenerative diseases known to be caused by the expansion of triplet repeat sequences in DNA, among them, Huntington's disease, many of the cerebellar ataxias, myotonic dystrophy, fragile-X syndrome, and Friedreich's ataxia; Friedreich's ataxia is the only autosomal recessive disorder in the group so far (the rest are autosomal dominant, except for fragile-X).[10] In Huntington's disease, we see anticipation only when the gene expansion is passed from the father to a child. The reverse is true for myotonic dystrophy. The congenital form occurs only when the myotonic dystrophy expansion originates from an affected mother. In both disorders, the sex of the affected offspring is irrelevant; that is, boys and girls are affected equally frequently.

Numerous models have been proposed to explain how the expansion of triplet repeats leads to human disease. At the DNA level, expansions in one of the two alleles can cause misalignment at meiosis, resulting in both deletions and further expansions. As a result, sometimes the gene can become completely disabled and fail to produce an mRNA transcript. These expansions can even have an effect on adjacent genes. When expanded segments are transcribed, the repeat triplets might affect protein folding and cause varying degrees of impairment of the action of the gene product.

III. Genomic Imprinting

In essence, the term **genomic imprinting** describes the differing phenotypes of some syndromes depending on the sex of the parent from whom the mutant allele is inherited. In other words, imprinted genes are expressed from only one chromosome in a parent-of-origin dependent manner. It is brought about by epigenetic instructions—imprints that are laid down in the parental germ cells. None of Mendel's experimental results predicted this phenomenon, since "hereditary factors" were transmitted to offspring without any sexual predilection.

mental patterning. Both sporadic and inherited mutations in the SHH gene cause holoprosencephaly. The color-coded pathway in Figure 1 of the paper by Villavicencio, Walterhouse, and Iannaconne[13] shows the additional anomalies, syndromes, and malignancies associated with malfunction of specific elements throughout the SHH cascade.

In addition, recent studies have shown that some congenital heart defects and cardiovascular anomalies result from mutations in transcription factors.[14] For example, mutations in NKX 2.5, a homeodomain transcription factor, cause familial congenital heart anomalies that include atrial septal defect (ASD), ventricular septal defect (VSD), and anomalies of the tricuspid valve (e.g., Ebstein's anomaly). The homeobox or homeopathic genes, first described in *Drosophila*, are so called because when mutated, they transform one of the insect's body segments into the likeness of another. A favorite illustration of the phenomenon is a fruit fly with a foot growing out of the head segment where an antenna should be.

One of the *Drosophila* homeobox transcription factors, **tinman**, a homolog of NKX 2.5, is expressed in the dorsal vessel, the insect equivalent of the vertebrate heart at the tube stage of development. Targeted disruption of tinman produces an absence of the dorsal vessel in *Drosophila*. A total of 10 NKX 2.5 mutations have been associated with familial congenital heart disease in humans, as mentioned above.

An exciting aspect of the discovery of these transcription factor mutations in relation to human disease is the potential for elucidating the complex processes of embryological development and eventually, the possibility of early detection and prevention of disease.

PEDIGREE DRAWING

Every new patient or family entering a practice of any kind merits at least a three-generation pedigree (Figure 1–11). Sometimes you will find indications from the initial screening family history that will indicate the necessity for a more detailed pursuit; for example, the need to concentrate on the maternal side in the case of an X-linked or possibly X-linked disease.

The three-generation screen will provide the ethnic origins of the families and should reveal any consanguinity. You might be surprised, however, to discover that the latter might not be mentioned until you specifically ask such a question as, "Are the two of you related other than by marriage?"

It is important to inquire about unexplained deaths, especially if at young ages, and note that infants or even children who died frequently get left out of the family history. Again, you have to ask specifically, "Were there any brothers or sisters who died?"

I usually write the surname across the bar between matings and put the country of origin or ethnic group in parentheses, as shown. The proband or

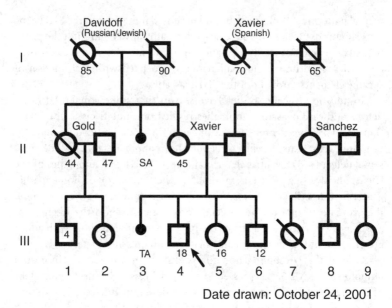

Figure 1–11 Three-generation pedigree. SA = spontaneous abortion; TA = therapeutic abortion.

index case, the individual who brought the family to your attention (and that is not necessarily the person affected with the condition), is marked with a diagonal arrow. The "grapes" hanging down among the siblings and labeled SA and TA represent spontaneous and therapeutic abortions, respectively. A diagonal line through the pedigree symbol means the individual is deceased.

Numbers written below the symbols usually represent the ages at the time the pedigree is drawn (always date the drawing) or the age at death. Numbers within the symbols are short-hand for numbers in a sibship. In generation III, for example, in the first branch at the left, there are four males and three females. To avoid having to give such directions as "first branch at the left," sometimes numbers are run consecutively from left to right below the symbols. Thus, each family member has a pedigree number. The proband, for example, becomes individual III-4; it's much easier to refer to specific individuals. If you decide to do the numbering that way, you'll have to figure out another way to indicate the ages to avoid confusion.

If your patient has a genetic disease or if there is one in the family, the person from whom you are obtaining the history might not be aware of the various manifestations. Thus, simply asking whether there are other affected individuals in the family might not work. You need to familiarize yourself with the condition and ask more specific questions. Consider, for example, osteogenesis imperfecta; obviously, you would ask if there are any relatives with unusually frequent fractures, but you need to know that in addition, a common manifestation of that connective tissue disorder is hyperflexible joints with or without recurring dislocations and poor teeth with unusually large numbers of cavities.

"Why bother with the routine three-generation pedigree?" I hear you ask. Well, aside from the obvious requirements above, you might be surprised at what you find out from family histories in cases of very common conditions. Heart disease and cancer are the conditions everyone is documenting these days. But consider a child with abdominal pain. If one of the parents or a sibling had proven appendicitis, that diagnosis moves higher up the list of possibilities.

Similarly, the siblings of a child with chronic otitis media should be considered as otitis prone and bear closer watching as fevers develop early in life. You ought to look a little harder for otitis as the cause and treat earlier and more aggressively. Attention to possible hearing loss and consideration of adenoidectomy earlier rather than later would be important issues to keep in mind.

The message is obvious: genetic predisposition plays a role in the majority of human illness. Positive family histories ought to raise your level of suspicion and help direct you to diagnostic tests, treatment, and preventive approaches.

WEB SITES

I do not see how it is possible for any physician to keep up to date without the Internet. In addition, the Web is probably the best way to familiarize yourself with the clinical manifestations of diseases, and the most appropriate diagnostic tests, treatment, and approaches to prevention. Already many of the best journals are on-line, as are key textbooks.

But caveats are in order. There is a great deal of misleading, if not totally wrong, information out there and every user, healthcare professional, or patient needs to learn how to search efficiently and how to select sites that are most likely to have data that are both current and reliable. There will be some trial and error, but a few simple guidelines will be helpful:

- Try to choose the sites of the well-known medical associations, such as the AMA, CMA, and the BMA and the specialty and subspecialty societies.
- Make a point of asking the experts in your field for their favorite Web sites when you see them at meetings, during consultations, or over coffee.
- When you use a Web site, use the same criteria for critical appraisal of data that you apply (or ought to apply) to journal articles.
- Web sites of support groups and specific disease organizations need to be recognized as possible two-edged swords. They might provide outstanding descriptions of diseases and be very useful to patients and families, particularly with day-to-day hints relating to management and coping

skills. A few, however, contain misinformation or such complex and potentially misleading material without a proper or interpretable context that they can cause more harm than good, especially when laypeople use them. If you plan to recommend one to a patient, check it out first yourself, and encourage your patients to bring questions and any areas of confusion to your attention. And be prepared for the patient who uncovers the latest advances before you do; it's a bit disconcerting at first—you'll soon learn to do a quick search of the recent literature the evening before you see any but the most routine patients.

Throughout this book, I refer to Web sites frequently, but to avoid the need to flip pages to find one when you've forgotten in which chapter you saw it, the following is a short list of those I visit most frequently and find most useful in relation to medical genetics.

1. Descriptions of Clinical Conditions

GeneClinics   <http://www.kumc.edu/gec/>
GeneTests   <http://www.genetests.org/>
If you think there might be a molecular or biochemical test for whatever disorder you suspect, try the GeneTests site. It will describe the test(s), which laboratory can run it, how to order it, and so on. It also has a directory of genetics counseling clinics in the United States and a link to GeneClinics.

Genetics in Primary Care   <http://genes-r-us.uthscsa.edu/resources/genetics/primary_care.htm>
Eight modules provide a series of teaching cases developed to be representative of patients seen in primary care that demonstrate genetic issues and principles. Each cites references, including Web sites and relevant consensus and policy statements. Topics include cardiovascular disease, colorectal cancer, developmental delay, and a separate module on ethical, legal, and social issues (ELSI). Overall—well done and worth perusing.

OMIM   <www3.ncbi.nlm.nih.gov/omim/searchomim.html>
This is the Online Mendelian Inheritance in Man, the famous catalog initiated by Victor A. McKusick in 1966. It contains descriptions, usually meticulously detailed, of single-gene disorders and often very useful descriptions of complex disorders. It's even useful for generating differential diagnoses by entering specific physical findings and obtaining a list of conditions in which that finding occurs.

NCHPEG   <http://www.nchpeg.org/>
This is the site for the National Coalition for Health Professional Education in Genetics. The coalition is made up of more than 100 organizations, including the AMA, CMA, BMA, ANA, and most of the genetics societies. It

is a fast-developing site for information on educational and clinical data in medical genetics and links to a wide variety of important sites, including those on this list.

Cancer genetics   <http://cancernet.nci.nih.gov/clinpdq/cancer_genetics/cancer>
The site contains much useful information on the genetic aspects of many types of cancer, describing who in a family is at risk, who ought to consider gene testing, and so on.

Mitochondrial disorders
United Mitochondrial Disease Foundation   <www.umdf.org>
Muscular Dystrophy Association   <www.mdausa.org/publications/Quest/q64mito.html>

Chromosome anomalies
GeneClinics   <http://www.kumc.edu/gec/>
Click on "Genetic Conditions" and then on "Chromosome Anomalies"

2. Teratology

Organization of Teratology Information Services (OTIS)
<http://www.otispregnancy.org/>
A compendium of teratology services in the United States and Canada.

Motherisk   <http://www.motherisk.org/>
One of the best sites for up-to-the-minute data on teratogens in pregnancy, effects of drugs during lactation, and other issues relevant to exposures to potentially toxic agents during pregnancy.

3. Genetics Societies

ASHG   <http://www.faseb.org/ashg/ashg.menu.htm>
The American Society of Human Genetics site provides useful links to a wide variety of reliable information, as well as a list of policy statements on such issues as genetic testing of children, newborn screening, and so on.

CCMG   <http://ccmg.medical.org/>
The Canadian College of Medical Geneticists

4. Genetics Support Groups

Genetic Alliance   <http://www.geneticalliance.org/>

A list of the support groups for genetic disorders in the United States and many other countries, including contact links.

Canadian Directory   <http://www.lhsc.on.ca/programs/medgenet/support.htm>

NORD   <http://www.rarediseases.org/>
If you don't find the organization you're seeking at the above sites, try the National Organization for Rare Diseases.

References

1. Dipple KM, McCabe RB. Phenotypes of patients with "simple" mendelian disorders are complex traits: thresholds, modifiers, and systems dynamics. Am J Hum Genet 2000;66:1729–35.
2. Willing MC, Deschenes SP, Scott DA, et al. Osteogenesis imperfecta type I: molecular heterogeneity for COL1A1 null alleles of type I collagen. Am J Hum Genet 1994;55:638–47.
3. Jegalian K, Lahn BT. Why the Y. Sci Am 2001;284:56–61.
4. Wallace DC. Mitochondrial DNA variation in human evolution, degenerative disease, and aging. Am J Hum Genet 1995;57:201–23.
5. Chinnery PF, Turnbull DM. Mitochondrial DNA mutations in the pathogenesis of human disease. Mol Med Today 2000;11:425–32.
6. Avner P, Heard E. X-chromosome inactivation: Counting, choice and initiation. Nat Rev Genet 2001;2:59–67.
7. Brown CJ, Robinson WP. The causes and consequences of random and non-random X chromosome inactivation in humans. Clin Genet 2000;58:353–63.
8. Stevenson DK, Verter J, Fanaroff AA, et al. Sex differences in outcomes of very low birth weight infants: the newborn male disadvantage. Arch Dis Child Fetal Neonatal Ed 2000;83:F182–5.
9. Harper PS, Harley HG, Reardon W, et al. Anticipation in myotonic dystrophy: New light on an old problem. Am J Hum Genet 1992;51:10–6.
10. Cummings CJ, Zoghbi HY. Fourteen and counting: unraveling trinucleotide repeat diseases. Hum Mol Genet 2000;9:909–16.
11. Riek W, Walters J. Genomic imprinting: parental influence on the genome. Nat Rev 2001;2:21–32.
12. Jones KL. Smith's recognizable patterns of human malformations. 6th ed. Fletcher J, ed. Philadelphia: WB Saunders; 1996.
13. Villavicencio EH, Walterhouse DO, Iannaccone PM. The Sonic hedgehog—patched—Gli pathway in human development and disease. Am J Hum Genet 2000;67:1047–54.
14. Benson D. Advances in cardiovascular genetics and embryology: role of transcription factors in congenital heart disease. Curr Opin Pediat 2000;12:497–500.

Complex Genetic Disorders: Alzheimer's Disease, Psychiatric Disorders, and Breast and Ovarian Cancer

Clinical Scenario

Dr. William Jones arrived at his office early on a Monday morning to check the weekend accumulation of e-mail. One was from Emily Johnston, a 50-year-old woman and a patient for more than 25 years. She was letting him know that her sister, age 55, had just been diagnosed as having Alzheimer's Disease. Although she hadn't mentioned it when Dr. Jones took the family history originally, in retrospect she is now concerned about the possibility that her father had the same manifestations at about the same age or maybe even earlier. He was becoming forgetful in his early 50s, to the point that he couldn't manage the family hardware business. For example, he would order goods that were already adequately stocked and would become almost belligerent when his wife would, as tactfully as she could, point this out to him. She was in the process of taking over most of the running of the store when he died of a heart attack at age 58.

Emily, calm and organized as usual, ended her letter as follows:

- *What is my risk of developing Alzheimer's disease?*
- *Is there DNA testing available? I'm sure I've seen something in a magazine but I didn't pay much attention at the time.*
- *What about the boys—what should I be telling them? John's just had his 30th birthday and Joe is 27. Both have "significant others" but neither has children.*

No sooner did Dr. Jones get though the weekend e-mail when the phone rang. It wasn't even 8 o'clock yet but on the line was George Merrill, one of the .com multimillionaires and a golf buddy of the doctor. "Willie, my lad, I need your advice. No, my golf swing is beyond repair; this is medical. No, we don't have a family doc; Margie and I are healthy and we just never got around to signing up with anybody; you'll do fine! We've had a bad weekend—my sister and I had to put our 75-year-old father in a seniors' retirement village. A major attraction of the place is their special facilities for Alzheimer's patients. That's what they told us Dad has. Now, I want that new gene testing stuff right away to make sure that's really what Dad has and to find out if I'm going to get it. Margie wants the test too and by the way, she's about three months pregnant...so what about this prenatal testing? If that's out there, we want that too...and right away! It doesn't matter how much it costs or where we have to go to get it."

Pause for a moment and write down what you think are the most important issues that the scenarios raise.

Your list ought to include at least the following:

- How likely is it that the diagnosis of Alzheimer's disease is correct?
- What are the manifestations of the disease?
- What conditions make up the differential diagnosis?
- What is a complex genetic disease and is Alzheimer's disease an example?
- Are there different types of Alzheimer's disease?
- What is known about the molecular genetics, and is testing clinically available?

Since this is a book on medical genetics, let's start with the genetic aspects.

COMPLEX DISEASES

1. What Are Complex Diseases?

It is now clear that the majority of human disorders fall into this category of conditions, which includes atherosclerotic heart disease, most congenital anomalies, most types of cancer, the psychiatric diseases, and even infections. (Isn't an infectious disease usually the result of a battle between two genomes, that of the host and that of the invading organism, each of which has opportunities for variability?) Some might even suggest that accidents and the injuries resulting from them have genetic components. Since we as humans lack the genes that specify a protective carapace like that of a tortoise, we are injury prone, and if one gives credence to the possibility of the existence of gene products in human populations that play a role in risk-taking behaviors, therein lies another predisposing genetic factor!

2. Complex versus Multifactorial

The term **multifactorial** has been used for traits presumably caused by more than one predisposing gene, with or without environmental factors, but is being replaced by the more comprehensive term, **complex**. **Multifactorial etiology** was the correct phrase, rather than the misleading **multifactorial heredity**, and it implied that there is more than one predisposing gene whose products, nearly always proteins, would interact with factors in the environment to overcome the homeostatic equilibrium of the organism. The end result: disease. (Homeostasis can be simply defined as the status quo: a steady state of lifelong stability of one's individuality in the face of the variety of experiences of a lifetime. It implies access to the environment, as well as protection from it, and it serves an evolutionary purpose, maintaining individuals as fit to reproduce; that is, it includes development—those devices that promote growth, differentiation, and maturation [Figure 2–1].) Complex disorders show familial aggregation without clear segregation, a key concept that tends to escape the casual observer. The *genes* of complex diseases segregate all right; it is the *phenotypes* that do not. The term **complex diseases** requires one to think not only about causative agents but also about physiological mechanisms that include evolution and developmental processes, all operating within specific societies and cultures. Complex diseases are more common than single-gene disorders and are the major contributors to morbidity and mortality in developed countries.

3. Single-Gene or Mendelian Traits As Complex Diseases

Having defined **complex**, it is essential to consider the fact that many mendelian single-gene diseases are really complex disorders in disguise. Individuals with, for example, glucose-6-phosphate dehydrogenase deficiency (see chapter 8, "Pharmacogenetics: Teratology"), an X-linked condition, might go through life without realizing that they have it if they never eat fava beans or are never exposed to the oxidizing drugs that precipitate hemolysis. Similarly, the autosomal recessive metabolic disease, phenylketonuria is remarkably complex (Figure 2–2). Classically, it is due to absent hepatic phenylalanine hydroxylase activity (more than 400 mutant alleles have been identified at that gene locus), but it also can be caused by inherited deficiencies in the synthesis pathway of its vitamin B_4 cofactor, and some forms of the enzyme deficiency due to different mutations do not cause the manifestations of the disease at all, even though phenylalanine

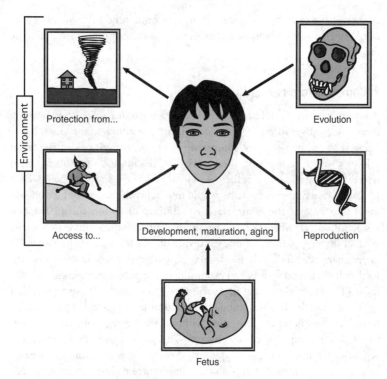

Figure 2–1 Elements of homeostasis.

levels in the blood are increased. Furthermore, the manifestations can be prevented by limiting phenylalanine intake in the diet, which is the therapy for the disease, and among infants and children with a phenylketonuria genotype in some Third World countries, there is no such disease phenotype as phenylketonuria because the protein intake in their meager diets is so low!

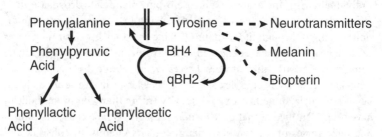

Figure 2–2 Metabolic pathways for phenylalanine, including the tetrahydrobiopterin cofactor. The block due to deficient phenylalanine hydroxylase activity is indicated by the double vertical lines.

chance that Emily's sister actually has Alzheimer's disease; that is, the diagnosis could be incorrect. Even if medical records indicate that the women's father probably had Alzheimer's disease, that's only two generations with affected individuals. Finally, it's unlikely that there would be any way to obtain DNA from the father for testing and thus, any mutation or variation found in the proband, Emily's sister, would be difficult to interpret. Nevertheless, a well-established mutant in the PSEN1 gene could be informative. The counseling ought to include the above data and caveats. Even if testing were available, would they wish it? And perhaps most importantly, research is continuing apace, and new diagnostic approaches will be developed, as might new approaches to treatment and prevention.

In a way, George Merrill's problems are more straightforward but probably will be more difficult to deal with. This is sporadic Alzheimer's disease, as far as can be determined, and DNA testing is not recommended, in spite of what the patient might have read or what Dr. Jones might find on the Internet, especially if either he or the patient get into the Web pages of some of the DNA and gene testing labs, which might be willing to do whatever test a patient or physician wishes as long as someone can pay for it! It would be a serious mistake to quote that old 2% to 3% without a long talk about why that number does not apply to an individual, and a referral to a genetics center would be almost mandatory in this situation. George will need to hear a consistent story from a couple of reliable sources before he will be able to make rational decisions and achieve some sort of peace.

PSYCHIATRIC DISORDERS

Schizophrenia and Manic-Depressive Affective Disorder

Schizophrenia is a severe and common psychiatric disorder affecting about 1% of the world's population. It is characterized by psychotic symptoms along with cognitive, affective, and psychosocial impairment. The only etiological factor that is firmly established is its heritability, and this is based on family, twin, and adoption studies. Nevertheless, the precise genetic mutations making up the genetic predisposition remain unknown. The situation is further confounded by the phenotypical heterogeneity, incomplete penetrance, and lack of a clear-cut pattern of inheritance.

Recently, diagnostic criteria have become more standardized so that schizophrenia is diagnosable from country to country with more confidence and consistency. There is, however, a broader phenotype known as the **spectrum disorders**, disease states that aggregate in families of schizophrenia patients but don't meet the criteria for the diagnosis of schizophrenia itself. There is, in addition, even some overlap with bipolar affective disorder; for example, relatives of schizoaffective patients show increased rates of schizophrenia, bipolar illness, and unipolar depression. Presumably there are shared susceptibility loci. Some linkage studies have shown several chromosome regions that are implicated in both schizophrenia and the bipolar disorders. Perhaps this should not be surprising in that both conditions have about the same prevalence in populations around the world, both show equal sex distributions, and both result from complex interactions between a variety of predisposing mutations and environmental and developmental factors.

As implied above, multiple candidate regions have been identified for the susceptibility loci in the human genome as possible sites but not all studies agree. At this time no molecular tests are available for either of these two conditions or their related variants.

Pervasive Developmental Disorders

Pervasive developmental disorders (PDD) are a group of conditions, including autism, Asperger's syndrome, and others. There is an average prevalence of about one in 2,500 children. In addition, autism or autistic behavior occurs with significantly increased frequency in a number of genetic conditions, most notably fragile-X syndrome and tuberous sclerosis.

The relative rarity of familial cases of PDD initially cast doubt on the existence of an inherited component for this disorder at all. However, although familial cases are relatively rare, they are substantially more frequent than would be predicted to occur by chance. Several genomic screens of populations looking for susceptibility loci have demonstrated only modestly positive or negative linkage evidence to date and there are no molecular tests available for the identification of children at risk.

Genetic Counseling

For the major psychiatric disorders, including schizophrenia, bipolar disease, severe depression, and PDD, the recurrence risks within families are low. The usual 2% to 5% figures apply but, as with all complex disorders, these are population risks and should be applied to an individual or to a family only after careful and detailed discussion.

BREAST AND OVARIAN CANCER

Breast and ovarian cancer are among the most complex of complex diseases. Let's deal primarily with breast cancer and mention some of the details on ovarian cancer in a separate section that follows.

First of all, what are the facts? The *lifetime* risk of breast cancer for women is one in eight or 12.5%, though that figure is distorted on the high side. It applies only at the time of birth and assumes that the population lives to 80 or more years. The risk of breast cancer rises with increasing age; for example, 80% of breast cancer occurs in women over age 50. Nevertheless, if a woman reaches age 50 without developing breast cancer, her chance of having breast cancer is some 10-fold *less* than one in eight simply because she's lived for five decades without developing it. In other words, there is an almost paradoxical decrease in risk as a woman becomes older even though the relative risk rises! In all, only 5% to 10% of breast cancer cases are familial.

Mutations in the *BRCA1* and *BRCA2* genes, discovered in 1994 and 1995, respectively, increase the risk of developing breast and ovarian cancer. For women with a mutation at either locus, the lifetime risk of acquiring breast cancer, often bilateral, is 56% to 85%, and there is a 16% to 40% risk of ovarian cancer. Men with a *BRCA1* or *BRCA2* mutation have up to a 16% risk of developing prostate cancer, and with a *BRCA2* mutation, about a 6% risk of acquiring breast cancer. The frequency of *BRCA* mutations in the general population is about one in 833 women; there are several *hundred* different *BRCA* mutations known at this time. Since the discovery of the *BRCA* genes, there has been a debate about whether presymptomatic mutation testing will be beneficial, and if so, which women should be eligible for such testing. There is no undisputed breast or ovarian cancer prevention option (see below) for those women found to be at increased risk. Therefore, the relatively low prevalence of the *BRCA* mutations, along with the absence of any good prevention program, leads us to conclude that general population screening for such mutants is unfeasible, both technically and financially, and therefore, undesirable. The American Society for Clinical Oncology recommends that testing be restricted to women at high risk of developing breast or ovarian cancer. Increased risk is indicated by a strong positive family history of one or both forms of cancer.

What constitutes a strong positive family history? There must be a close family member on the mother's or father's side known to have had breast cancer. Breast cancer in men is rare but obviously, fathers have sisters, a mother, aunts, and grandmothers. A close family member is defined as a parent, sibling, aunt, uncle, or grandparent on either side. Early onset (before age 40) also increases the chance of a cancer being familial. In addition, the presence of ovarian cancer in the family increases the risk of a *BRCA* mutation significantly.

Not all familial breast cancer is associated with *BRCA* mutations; there are undoubtedly other loci involved in the predisposition to breast cancer. Many environmental and lifestyle factors have been proposed; none has been clearly supported by evidence. Breast size and trauma are not factors, nor is the use of oral contraception. The jury is still out on high-fat diets, estrogen replacement therapy during and postmenopause, alcohol, and cigarette smoke.

Ethnic Population Screening

Are there populations in which an increased incidence of breast or ovarian cancer makes screening on a population basis less inhibitory? Among the Ashkenazi Jews, the *BRCA1* mutations 185delAG and 5382insC and the *BRCA2* mutation 6174delT are seen with increased frequencies, probably as a result of founder effect. Slightly more than 2% of Ashkenazi Jewish women carry one of these three mutations (as compared to the general population prevalence of one in 833 women for any *BRCA* mutation); tests are commercially available but the question remains: Is screening indicated for specific populations rather than just those with positive family histories? The answer is not straightforward and further research is needed.

Risks for breast cancer conferred by any of the three mutations are about 50% by age 50 years and about 85% by age 70. If we combine this penetrance with the prevalence of the 185delAG mutation in *BRCA1* among Ashkenazi Jews, theoretically the prediction would be that about 19% of Jewish women with breast cancer by age 50 and about 9% by age 70 will be carriers of one of those mutations. Thus, up to 40% of all Ashkenazi Jewish breast cancer patients aged less than 50 could be carriers of the known founder mutations in *BRCA1* and *BRCA2*.

Other populations are similarly affected. In the Icelandic population, *BRCA2* 999del5 is seen with increased frequency, undoubtedly as a result of founder effect. Therefore, it would *seem* that there is a sound rationale for screening of the Ashkenazi Jewish and Icelandic populations. However, actual studies on these populations have demonstrated considerably smaller incidence figures than those above.

So what is our bottom line? All women are at high risk for breast cancer and the ever-changing recommendations for surveillance must be monitored by all physicians who provide health care for women. General population screening for *BRCA* mutations is not indicated, but screening for *BRCA* mutations in an affected individual with a positive family history is an option, especially if the ages of onset tend to be less than 40 years. Ethnic screening, currently confined to Ashkenazi Jews and the Icelandic population, remains an issue to be sorted out by research.

All of the above information is subject to change and reinterpretation on the basis of research; referral for consultation is essential (see "Caveats" below).

Management of Presymptomatic Individuals With *BRCA* Mutations

Herein lies the problem: there is no technique or approach that offers 100% prevention. The value of drugs, including tamoxifen, in reducing the chance of developing breast cancer in high-risk women is not established. Surveillance by periodic mammograms starting at age 35 has been suggested, but

- To present the relatively few laboratory procedures most likely to provide diagnostic clues
- To describe methods for putting together the elicited data in order to maximize the chances of reaching a diagnosis
- To provide a general management plan for the patient and family regardless of whether a specific diagnosis is reached
- To provide guidelines for genetic counseling

How Common Are Birth Defects?

The incidence of birth defects depends on when you look. At birth, the most usually quoted number is 3%. That sounds small, but if you are delivering babies in your practice, keep in mind that about one of every 30 babies will have a potentially serious congenital anomaly! A congenital heart defect, for example, is found in just under one of every 100 live births.

Obviously, not every congenital anomaly will be detected at birth. Pyloric stenosis doesn't become manifest until the affected infant is 6 weeks old on average, many major anomalies of the brain are silent until developmental delays are noted or seizures begin, abnormal teeth won't show up until the teeth erupt (or fail to erupt on time), and so on. Surveys at age 7 years indicate an 8% to 9% prevalence of at least one major malformation and congenital anomalies are among the three major causes of morbidity and mortality in infants and children, accidents and cancer being the other two.

By the way, the word **congenital** simply means present at birth. Although most isolated anomalies and syndromes have a genetic component, as discussed in the next section, the term has no etiological connotation. Intrauterine infections, for example, can cause congenital malformations. As already noted, detection of anomalies actually *present* at birth can be delayed for weeks to years for a variety of reasons. And speaking of definitions, how about **incidence** and **prevalence**? See if you can explain the difference and then check the glossary.

Classification of Congenital Anomalies

There are many ways of categorizing malformations, such as by cause, by organ(s) affected, or by developmental process (agenesis, hypoplasia). The one that is most widely used by dysmorphologists, mainly because it is actually helpful, is the following:

Malformation

A malformation is a structural defect of any part of the organism due to an intrinsically abnormal developmental process. "Intrinsically" implies that the defect was present from conception or early embryonic life and is likely to be

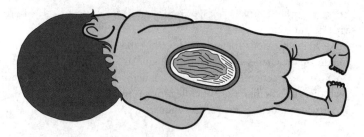

Figure 3–2 Neural tube defect (meningocele)—a malformation.

genetic, but not necessarily. Figure 3–2 shows a typical example, a neural tube defect.

Deformation

A deformation is an abnormal form, shape, or position of a part of the body caused by mechanical forces; for example, oligohydramnios for any reason can cause clubfeet, dislocation of the hip, and flattening of facial features simply because the fetus is jammed up against the uterine wall rather than floating freely. Figure 3–3 depicts an infant with renal agenesis (Potter's syndrome), showing the flattened face and deformed feet.

Disruption

A disruption is a structural defect due to extrinsic breakdown of or interference with an originally normal developmental process. Teratogens fit in

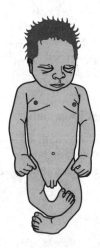

Figure 3–3 Potter's syndrome—a deformation. Note the flattened facial features and the abnormal positioning of the feet.

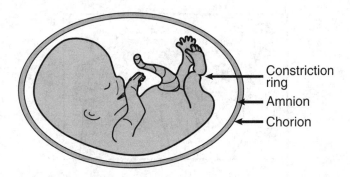

Figure 3–4 Constriction ring due to amniotic band—a disruption.

here, as do amputations of limbs as a result of amniotic bands (Figure 3–4 shows a typical constriction ring due to an amniotic band) or the so-called vascular disruption syndromes (e.g., Poland's syndrome). Although strictly speaking disruptions should not be genetic and therefore familial cases are rare, there could be predisposing genes in the initiating event; for example, the severity of the effects of alcohol on a fetus depends to some extent on the genome of the mother and the fetus.

Dysplasia

Dysplasia is an abnormal organization of cells into tissue(s). The connective tissue diseases and many of the bone dysplasias are examples.

Recognition of the category into which a defect best fits can be helpful in determining its etiology.

Importance of Syndrome Recognition

Some might look on syndrome diagnosis as a sort of intellectual game played among consultants and trainees on rounds so that the players can demonstrate how clever they are (Figure 3–5). Nothing could be farther from the truth. Think back to the clinical scenario and have a look now at the reasons you wrote down for bothering to go through the admittedly often complex series of events that may or may not get you to the correct cause and correct diagnosis (in addition to getting the family into the proper support group!). Here they are:

1. **Prognosis.** Is the patient likely to survive; is there associated mental retardation and if so, how severe; and are there other anomalies that might not be obvious on physical examination or that might develop later in life?
2. **Management.** Are there early interventions that could prevent complications (a compelling example is Beckwith-Wiedemann syndrome, in

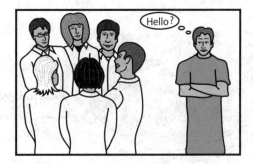

Figure 3–5 Syndrome rounds.

which hypoglycemia is a frequent occurrence in the neonatal period and if untreated, permanent brain damage can occur), is corrective surgery available and how good is it, and are there measures to be taken to minimize risks for future children (e.g., avoidance of alcohol, taking folate supplements for prevention of neural tube defects)?

3. **Genetic counseling**. If you get the diagnosis wrong, you might give the family an incorrect recurrence risk for future affected children and the wrong risks for other relatives within the family.

And finally, before we go on, a caveat: do not be discouraged by the oft-quoted figures indicating that 30% to 60% of infants with various constellations of birth defects do not receive a specific diagnosis no matter how many super-specialists they see. Those numbers come mostly from genetics clinics; by the time patients get to those centers, they already have been seen by competent physicians, often including experienced pediatricians, and if those specialists have failed to recognize a syndrome, obviously there is a reduced chance that one can be discerned. Those syndromes diagnosed without referral or prior to referral for management and counseling don't get included in the stats. Your batting average will be higher.

Having said this, it should be emphasized that all individuals with malformation syndromes should be assessed in a center where there will be a team of experts prepared to deal with the many complex issues that can emerge.

SYNDROME-ORIENTED PHYSICAL EXAMINATION

Since the first encounter with the patient is often in the delivery room or newborn nursery, the examination may occur before a detailed history is obtained. So let's break precedence and start with the physical examination. Keep in mind that the primary objective is to distinguish what is normal from what is abnormal. Failure to recognize minor (and sometimes not so minor!) anomalies frequently accounts for the failure to make a diagnosis. Even the most sophisticated computer cannot (at least as yet !) do an examination for you.

1. Look. First *look*, don't touch.
   - Facial features. Assess the facial features before the infant starts to cry.
   - Look at the patient from different angles. It's surprisingly easy to miss cranial asymmetry unless you squat down at the end of whatever the infant is lying on and observe (Figure 3–6). Similarly, look carefully at the undressed and undiapered patient for asymmetry of the limbs and the body in general. Check body proportions: do the limbs and head size appear to be right for the body size?
   - Moving parts. Does the baby move the limbs and head. Guess what—if a humerus is fractured during labor or delivery, the neonate won't be moving that arm very often!

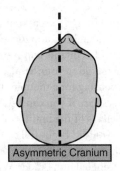

Asymmetric Cranium

Figure 3–6 An easy-to-miss physical finding: asymmetry.

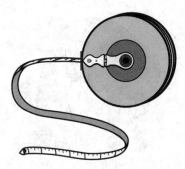

Figure 3–7 The tape measure—don't leave home without it!

2. Measure. If I were to take away all your instruments but one, which should you be most anxious to keep? As in Figure 3–7, no question—the tape measure.

   Time to touch:

   • Head size. *Never* omit this measurement from the examination of a newborn and in follow-up examinations and *always*, of course, relate it to body length and weight. By the time hydrocephalus becomes obvious, it might be too late to intervene and prevent brain damage.

   • Don't trust your memory—plot the data on the appropriate growth charts. There are charts for upper to lower body segments, intercanthal distances, fontanelle sizes, palpebral fissure lengths, and even length of fingers in relation to length of palm. Some of the more important are included among the references and further reading for this chapter; others are available from a clinical guideline to congenital malformations from the New York State Department of Health (nysdoh) (see "Comments" on Web sites) and in the *Handbook of Normal Physical Measurements*.[1]

3. Muscle tone. This is something to keep in mind as you do your examination. Obviously, limbs shouldn't flop loosely; learn to appreciate the differences in head control as infants mature, and *always* pick a baby up by the armpits, and then hold in your hand, as shown in Figure 3–8, to assess tone. It's worth pausing for a moment to think about hypotonia. What are its main causes? See if you can list at least three before going on. If you got severe defects of the brain, chromosome anomalies, and spinal muscle atrophy, you did beautifully. Obviously, there are a host of syndromes in which hypotonia can be a prominent feature but one in particular should be singled out, Prader-Willi syndrome. The typical

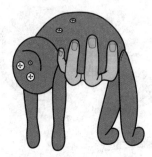

Figure 3–8 The **floppy baby**. Congenital hypotonia is easy to miss if you don't pick an infant up.

signs (see Glossary) will not be present at birth or even over the early months of life, but any newborn with profound hypotonia without an obvious cause must have, in addition to a regular karyotype, a fluorescent in-situ hybridization (FISH) examination to check for a deletion in chromosome 15q.

4. The cry. If the baby doesn't cry at some time during your examination, do not complete your assessment until you've heard the "voice." Flicking the bottom of the foot is a humane way to elicit crying. What you're listening for are such things as the high-pitched cry of a brain-damaged infant, the low-pitched, almost growly, cry of the infant with hypothyroidism or Hurler's syndrome and, needless to say for the budding syndromologist, the mewing kitten-like cry of the patient with cri du chat syndrome (yes, it really does sound like a kitten mewing!).

General Physical Examination

The following are just some areas and features to be given special attention when looking for some of the more subtle anomalies that could be extremely important in coming to a syndrome diagnosis. Clearly, a careful systematic examination is essential. However, what we're trying to do here is create a list of all the major and minor anomalies in order to maximize the chance of getting to the most likely diagnosis.

Head and Neck

The fontanelles are clues to the presence of micro- and hydrocephaly (Figure 3–9). Look for any unusual shape of the cranium and the facial structures, such as brachycephaly or flattened facies. Before deciding whether the facial appearance is "odd," look carefully at the parents' faces.

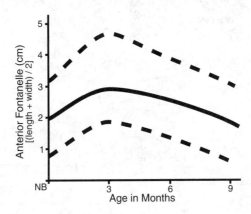

Figure 3–9 Chart depicting anterior fontanelle measurements over the first nine months.

Eyes. You really do have to open them up, even in a newborn, if only to be certain they are present and of normal size. Watch for lid anomalies, such as ptosis or notching, and the presence of eyelashes and eyebrows. Do you know what synophrys is and when it is seen normally? It means eyebrows that meet in the midline, and it is seen commonly in many dark-skinned races and ethic groups, including Arabs and East Indians. Synophrys is also a sign found in several syndromes, for example, Cornelia de Lange's syndrome. Now, see if you can sketch the typical **epicanthal fold** seen in Down syndrome (Figure 3–10). Colobomas or gaps in the iris (Figure 3–11) can be difficult to see in an infant—be sure you have a good light source. The coloboma, if confined to the iris, causes no impairment of vision but it can extend posteriorly and cause defects of the choroid, retina, and even the optic nerve with variable degrees of blindness.

Ears. Determining whether they are low set depends on getting the head properly oriented, as illustrated in Figure 3–12. Keep the embryology in mind. The external ear develops from nodules on the first and second branchial arches in the upper neck region; the first cleft gives rise to the ear canals and eustachian tubes. As the ear develops, it ascends and tilts anteriorly; thus, an ear that appears low set and is also posteriorly tilted is more likely to be truly low set. If in doubt, don't include it as a positive physical sign.

The complicated drawings of the external ear in the anatomy books aren't worth memorizing; the three-line drawing, as shown in Figure 3–13, is fine for most of the anomalies you need to recognize. Any variation of the

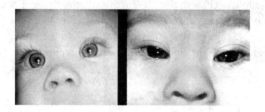

Figure 3–10 Epicanthal fold seen in Down syndrome.

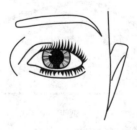

Figure 3–11 Coloboma: you'll never see it if you don't get the infant's eyes open.

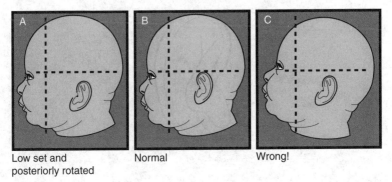

Low set and   Normal   Wrong!
posteriorly rotated

Figure 3–12 Assessing the low-set ear. In *A* and *B*, the head is correctly oriented with the eyes looking straight ahead. With the head tilted as in *C*, the examiner may incorrectly interpret the ears as low set.

major landmarks should be noted and counted as one of the anomalies in your final assessment, even something as tricky to pick up as absence of the anterior crus of the antihelix. Occasionally a minor ear variant, such as the latter, will cause a computer-assisted diagnosis program to include a syndrome or group of syndromes in which an ear anomaly is almost always found and which might have been omitted from the list of diagnostic possibilities without it.

Referring again to the embryology, it will not be a big surprise to realize that anomalous external ears can be a warning flag of impaired hearing due to anomalous development of the ear canal or other internal auditory structures. The sooner hearing deficits are discovered, the better the prognosis for normal intellectual and psychosocial development of the child.

And one last item: ear creases (Figure 3–14). Can you think of a condition in which creases in the lobes are present? (see *ear creases* in the glossary).

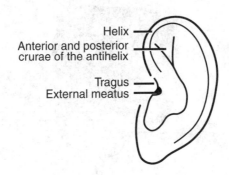

Helix
Anterior and posterior
crurae of the antihelix

Tragus
External meatus

Figure 3–13 The external ear (auricle) showing just the major landmarks.

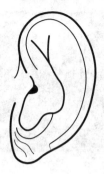

Figure 3–14 Earlobe creases.

Nose. Note the size in relation to the face as well as any unusual shapes. Some examples of abnormal noses are diagrammed in Figures 3–15 and 3–16.

Mouth. Again, is it too big or too small for the face? Do you remember what the philtrum is?

Open the child's mouth and check the alveolar ridges. Enlargement can be a sign of a storage disease (gangliosidosis, mucopolysaccharidosis) but the most common cause in the older infant or child is poor tongue thrust secondary to hypotonia from any cause.

When the patient is old enough to have teeth, for heaven's sake, take a look at them! They are a frequent source of diagnostic clues but are often overlooked. Note the number, spacing, shape, and condition and quality of the enamel. Describe what you see in Figure 3–17. What condition(s) might this be? (see *teeth* in the glossary). Also keep in mind that some 20% of humans, that's one in five, have missing or extra teeth and most of the time the numerical anomalies are dominantly inherited, although there is often

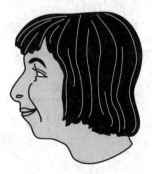

Figure 3–15 The beaked nose of Rubinstein-Taybi syndrome. Note the nasal septum protruding below the nares.

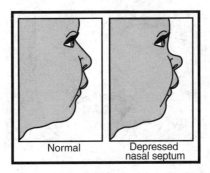

Figure 3–16 Saddle nose (depressed nasal septum).

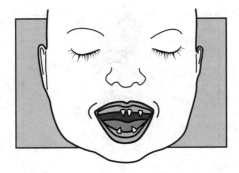

Figure 3–17 Conical teeth.

considerable intrafamilial variability. What about a single central upper incisor? Believe it or not, it's a sign of holoprosencephaly.

Tongue. A normal infant does not keep its mouth open for very long, and if you see an open-mouthed neonate, what would you think of? Either the muscle tone is so bad that the jaw simply falls open or the tongue is too big to fit into the oral cavity. See if you can come up with some conditions characterized by macroglossia. Sometimes an abnormally shaped tongue can provide a diagnostic clue, as in Figure 3–18. Of course, once in a while a normal-sized tongue might overfill an oral cavity that is too small.

Jaw. You can miss micrognathia if you don't take the time to look at the head in profile.

Neck. Watch for webbing (Figure 3–19) or redundant skin folds, low hairline, and a neck that is too short. What might appear as unusually sloping

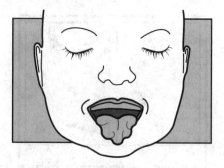

Figure 3–18 Lobulated tongue seen in, for example, some of the oral-facial-digital syndromes.

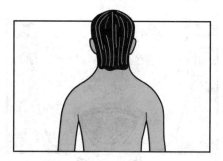

Figure 3–19 Webbed neck and sloped shoulders.

shoulders, as in the illustration, could in fact be caused by webbing of the neck.

Chest, Back, and Abdomen

Check for pectus excavatum (caved-in) or carinatum (protruding or pigeon breast). Note other configurations of the chest; for example, a small, bell-shaped chest is suggestive of skeletal dysplasia (Figure 3–20). An unusually short sternum is seen commonly in which chromosome anomaly (see glossary)?

Be sure that the nipples are present (they could be hypoplastic or even totally absent in ectodermal dysplasia) and that there are only two! If you are concerned about the possibility that the nipples are widely spaced, you can measure the internipple distance in relation to the chest circumference and check it on the appropriate chart.

Scoliosis is easy to miss; if you see it or suspect it, order X-rays. If the scoliosis is due to anatomical anomalies of vertebrae, you have a potentially diagnostic finding to list.

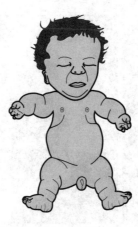

Figure 3–20 Severe bone dysplasia syndrome with bell-shaped tiny thorax and short limbs.

Check the quality of abdominal muscles and for hernias, organomegaly, and masses. Wilms' tumor and neuroblastoma are not the most common causes of abdominal masses in infants. So, what is? Renal anomalies.

Count the umbilical vessels. Now that the dust has settled, the notion of a single umbilical artery (SUA), that is, a two-vessel cord, as a signpost for kidney anomalies is arguable. However, an infant with a two-vessel cord has about a seven-fold greater risk of having additional malformations, the most common being cardiac. In addition, SUA is seen frequently in trisomies 18 and 13. Treat it as an anomaly that, like most anomalies, is reason enough to search carefully for others. SUA is frequently detected on fetal ultrasonograms and some would recommend a fetal karyotype even if no other anomalies are found. In any event, it is an indication for very careful additional fetal ultrasonography and a follow-up of the pregnancy. A reasonable course to follow is that if after the 22- or 23-week ultrasonogram no other anomaly besides the SUA is found, a karyotype is not indicated.

Limbs

Short limbs. Where is the major shortening, proximal (rhizomelia, rhizo meaning "root") or distal (acromelia); mesomelia indicates generalized shortening.

Long limbs. If the limbs appear too long, do an upper segment to lower segment ratio (the dividing point is the upper border of the pubic symphysis) and check the result on the chart. Manifestations of Marfan syndrome can be present at birth.

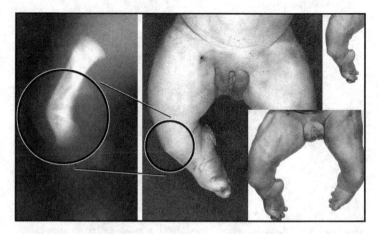

Figure 3–21 Camptomelia (bent limb).

Bent limbs. Bowing of the limbs (also known as "knock knees") are seen in a variety of syndromes, usually with short stature. Figure 3–21 shows a characteristic sign of the often lethal but highly variable bent-limb conditions known as camptomelia. Frequently there is a skin dimple over the bend.

Bony aplasias. It is easy to forget to check for the presence of the ulna, the fibula, and the patella; the absence or hypoplasia of any of which might be a diagnostic clue, especially when other bone anomalies are present or suspected. Can you name a syndrome in which the absence of the radius with or without anomalies of the thumb is seen? High marks for thinking of Fanconi's anemia! Although not strictly a part of the limb, don't miss absence or hypoplasia of the clavicles, as in cleidocranial dysostosis.

Hands

Size. Are the hands unusually small or short? Again, there are tables to consult. Are they pudgy, as in Coffin-Lowry syndrome, or do they look that way because of dorsal lymphedema (a sign of Turner's syndrome in the neonate).

Finger shape. Are they long and thin as seen in Marfan syndrome? Is there clinodactyly or camptodactyly (deflected or bent finger), usually referring to the 5th finger, as in Figure 3–22, but also seen with camptomelia affecting other fingers and toes.

   Polydactyly can occur as an isolated anomaly, often inherited as an autosomal dominant trait, or as one manifestation of several syndromes. It *must* be noted as being preaxial or postaxial. Think of the hand at the side with the

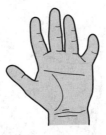

Figure 3–22 Hand showing a short 5th finger with clinodactyly (bent finger). Note also a single transverse palmar crease.

palms flat on the thigh—preaxial is anterior and thus it would be the thumb involved in a partial or total duplication; postaxial polydactyly is duplication of part or all of the 5th finger. Even a barely visible skin tag counts as polydactyly—look carefully for that one. In fact, it is easier than you might think to miss polydactyly, especially postaxial, in an aborted fetus, stillbirth, or even full-term infant. Do a count; it only takes a couple of seconds!

Fifth finger. Figure 3–22 shows a typical short 5th finger with only two phalanges and a single crease, as seen in Down syndrome. This is due to aplasia or severe hypoplasia of the middle phalanx. Curiously, the short, usually bent, 5th digit with either a single crease or the two creases very close together is probably the most common congenital anomaly associated with a chromosomal defect!

Distal fat pads. If the distal fat pads are almost pointed, as in Figure 3–23, that is, there is persistence of the fetal fat pads, you might have a clue to the possibility of Kabuki syndrome.

Thumb. Note its presence, hypoplasia, or absence, as well as shape and number of segments; for this digit, three segments is abnormal. An easy-to-

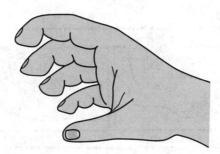

Figure 3–23 Persistent fetal fat pads.

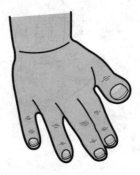

Figure 3–24 Broad thumb.

miss feature is the point of insertion of the thumb in relation to the wrist: is it too far proximal or too distal? Also note its size; shown in Figure 3–24 is the typical broad thumb seen in Rubinstein-Taybi syndrome. Once in a while you will see an adducted thumb across the palm that is difficult to straighten, as seen, for example, in some of the arthrogryposis syndromes and trisomy 18.

Nails. Note the shape and size of the fingernails. Clubbed fingers *can* occur in a neonate. Toenails typically are quite variable and hard to assess. Hypoplastic to near-absent nails is the most distal, and can be the most subtle sign of, for example, anticonvulsant embryopathy; that is, if it's real, it counts as a **limb reduction defect**.

Feet

Most of the hand anomalies described above also can be seen in feet, but in addition, note the so-called rocker-bottom foot, typical of trisomy 18, illustrated in Figure 3–25. This is caused by a tilted talus. Varying degrees of

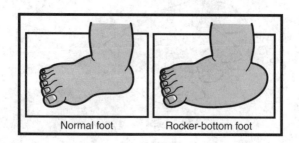

Normal foot   Rocker-bottom foot

Figure 3–25 Rocker-bottom feet with prominent heels.

clubfeet can occur as isolated defects, sometimes due to a positional deformation (remember those four types of congenital anomalies!) secondary to oligohydramnios—but it could be a syndrome manifestation and hence, a malformation.

Genitalia

Male. Check phallus size. A micropenis is seen in several syndromes; can you think of one in which a macropenis is present (see chapter 4, "Ambiguous Genitalia")? Make sure you identify the urethral orifice; if it is misplaced, check for additional anomalies, especially of the urogenital system. Finally, find *both* testes and familiarize yourself with their size and consistency.

Female. An apparently enlarged clitoris could indicate ambiguous genitalia, as can various degrees of fusion of the labia majora (Figure 3–26). An inguinal mass in the groin of an apparent female is unlikely to be an ovary! Be sure to locate the urethral, vaginal, and rectal orifices, and check for increased pigmentation.

A detailed approach to sexual differentiation is presented in chapter 4.

Skin

Pigment and vascular anomalies. Most lesions, including café-au-lait spots, nevi, hemangiomas, and so on, are obvious, but look carefully for *de*pigmented areas. Learn to recognize the normal variations of skin mottling, color, desquamation, and other apparent irregularities by observation of as many normal babies as you can examine.

Hair. Again, the variation is extraordinary. Observe the posterior hairline in normal infants so that you will be able to recognize when it might be low. Certain patterns might help you with syndrome diagnoses. Note the odd pattern of hair laterally onto the side of the face in a child with Treacher

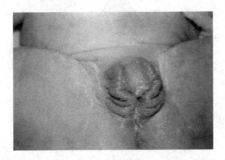

Figure 3–26 Masculinized female external genitalia.

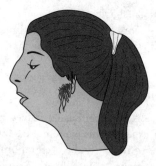

Figure 3–27 Treacher Collins syndrome. Note the hair growing anterior to the ear.

Collins syndrome in Figure 3–27 (some will not have the obvious ear abnormality to tip you off!).

This is a rather long list of checkpoints, more or less organized as for any physical examination. The American College of Medical Genetics guidelines (see Web site) include a list of headings that might serve as a reminder. I suggest making your own list, leaving off the items you're sure you cover all the time and emphasizing those you personally tend to miss or that were new to you.

SYNDROME-ORIENTED HISTORY

Pregnancy

Inquire about possible exposure to teratogens, for example, maternal infections, drugs, alcohol, or X-rays (Figure 3–28 and chapter 8, "Pharmacogenetics: Teratology"). Also ask about any prenatal testing, such as maternal serum screening. Be sensitive to the possibility of maternal guilt whenever there is a

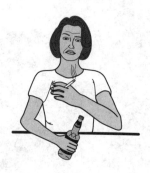

Figure 3–28 Some moms do, even today!

child with an anomaly. More often than not, the guilt will be unsupported by fact and it is extremely important to counsel and support the parents. For example, a drug taken during the third month of pregnancy could not possibly have caused a neural tube defect because the neural tube closes by 6 weeks' gestation and no external agent is likely to blow it open 6 weeks later!

On routine fetal ultrasonography, clues can appear as early as 10 to 14 weeks, when, for example, excess nuchal translucency in fetuses with Down syndrome, other trisomies, Turner's syndrome, and triploidy can be visualized (Figure 3–29). It is important to emphasize the indication for serial ultrasonography if any suspicious signs appear. The amount of amniotic fluid, for example, is significant. Keep in mind that throughout the latter half of pregnancy, most of the amniotic fluid is fetal urine, and amniotic fluid homeostasis demands intact fetal genitourinary and gastrointestinal tracts, as well as a functional brain stem that can control fetal swallowing.

The computer program PLATYPUS is an extensive, interactive prenatal ultrasonography reference and diagnostic tool providing access to current anatomical systems and procedures. It is available in many major hospitals and is designed mainly for the ultrasonographer but provides fascinating and useful data for the novice as well. For more information, the Web site is <www.firstsofware.com/Platypus.htm>.

Development

Learning the timing of the major developmental milestones is essential and they are well defined in every textbook of pediatrics. In addition, it is crucial to ascertain whether, for a developmentally delayed child, there was a period of time over which development was definitely normal. **Delays stemming from birth usually have etiologies that are very different from those starting at 6 months of age or later**. However, being certain that the parents

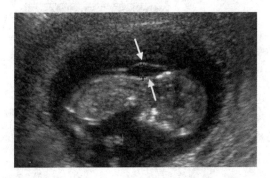

Figure 3–29 Fetal ultrasonogram, first trimester, showing excess nuchal translucency. (Picture courtesy of Dr. Ants Toi, Radiology, Mt. Sinai Hospital, University of Toronto.)

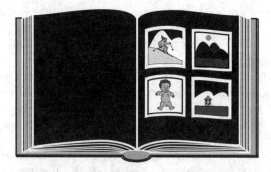

Figure 3–30 The family photograph album can be a treasure trove of valuable information.

are providing accurate data might not be so easy—there could be several siblings and the developmental histories tend to get mixed up, or the parents might not be capable of giving a good history for a variety of reasons, including their guilt over possibly having caused the birth defects or their own intellectual impairment.

There are some tricks! The family photograph album is one (Figure 3–30). For example, a snapshot of a child performing a task that he or she can no longer handle could be a major clue to the diagnosis of a neurodegenerative disease. In addition, many families document their children's development on videotape. And don't miss the opportunity to compare features of your patient with those of siblings, parents, and other relatives.

The schoolteacher (Figure 3–31) is an often-untapped source of knowledge of developmental data, intellect, and sometimes the later onset or loss of skills or changes in attention span that might initially go unnoticed by parents but might signal the onset of an inherited neurodegenerative disease.

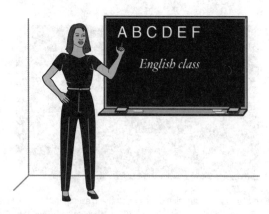

Figure 3–31 The school is a too-often-neglected source of data of both intellect and behavior.

Family History

The three-generation family history, as described in chapter 1, is usually sufficient, although the direction will be dictated by the emerging nature of the problem; for example, if the condition is X-linked, obviously the maternal side of the family would merit a closer look.

When the diagnosis is either established or highly suspected, the physician must familiarize him- or herself with the whole spectrum of manifestations, which is now quite easy to do using the various sources of syndrome descriptors described at the end of this chapter. There could be considerable *inter-* as well as the usual *intra*familial variability. For example, in families with the connective tissue disorder osteogenesis imperfecta (fragile-bone disease), some affected relatives might have had no fractures but manifest markedly hyperextensible joints.

The family picture album might again prove invaluable. I can recall being able to construct a relatively complete (no pun intended!) pedigree of Crouzon's disease (craniofacial dysostosis) from a wedding photograph. Frequently in families there will be a historian; all one has to do is find that person, most often a woman, usually a grandmother. The family Bible could be another source of important history (Figure 3–32).

Often it is essential to see and examine the parents and siblings; obviously this is so when familial conditions are possibilities. Do not fall into the trap of accepting the findings of colleagues who might not be as familiar with the condition in question as you have become.

And finally, beware of medical diagnoses provided by family members for their relatives. Whenever possible, obtain copies of the medical records (with signed release of information forms, of course). During the investigation of a family with familial polyposis with several affected siblings and

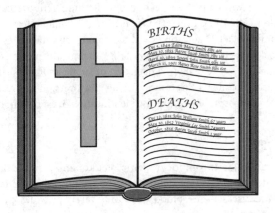

Figure 3–32 The family Bible may contain the most accurate family histories.

a mother who apparently also had the disease (long history of rectal bleeding; no suggestive history of familial polyposis on the husband's side), when we finally found the surgeon who had operated on her, it turned out that she had had hemorrhoids but no polyps. We had been issuing warnings to the wrong side of the family: the mother had run a boarding house and had carried on a long-standing affair with one of her boarders who, we soon discovered, had died of "bowel cancer" but not before fathering the three affected siblings!

LABORATORY INVESTIGATIONS

Diagnostic Imaging

For the undiagnosed infant with a congenital malformation, a total body X-ray is indicated, with special attention to any area that is malformed or asymmetrical. You will be surprised at how often a specific and unanticipated skeletal anomaly will provide you with an important clue to the diagnosis. Ultrasonography is also important for the soft-tissue defects and to at least begin the process of sorting out structural anomalies of the central nervous system. The ultrasonographer can usually get a good scan of the brain as long as the anterior fontanelle is open. Obviously, computed tomographic scans, magnetic resonance imaging, and echocardiography will be valuable when indicated.

Karyotype

Any patient with two or more anomalies and no diagnosis (or perhaps only one anomaly if there is developmental delay) should have a chromosome analysis as part of the work-up. New technology, including fluorescent in-situ hybridization (FISH)[4] and the expansion of that technique to simultaneous specific staining of all 22 autosomes and the X and Y chromosomes, each with a distinct color (spectral karyotyping or SKY),[5] has greatly increased the resolution of the analyses and allowed detection of subtle anomalies such as tiny deletions, small fragments, tiny translocations, and inversions. Increasing use of specific DNA probes is allowing precise identification of even point mutations.

Hematology

Although anemia, thrombocytopenia, leukopenia, and other blood dyscrasias do occur in some syndromes, they tend to develop later in the course of the disease; thus, blood work only rarely provides clues to syndrome diagnosis.

Metabolic Screening

This is a difficult issue. It is too often ordered as part of the routine investigation of a child with undiagnosed malformations, yet judicious use will provide diagnostic clues more frequently than advertised in older guidelines for diagnosis of syndromes. Although, for instance, signs of the mucopolysaccharidoses (MPS), such as Hurler's syndrome, are rarely congenital, an MPS screen is the essential first step in the diagnostic work-up. Most of the classic inborn errors of metabolism, examples being phenylketonuria and galactosemia, are not characterized by malformations (congenital cataracts *do* occur in some newborns with galactosemia). Recent studies have been expanding the borders of the inborn errors. Smith-Lemli-Opitz syndrome, for example, consisting of a constellation of malformations, is now known to be associated with a defect in steroid biosynthesis.

Mitochondrial Diseases

These are rare causes of congenital anomalies but keep the possibility in mind when you see unusual combinations of such traits as hearing loss with cardiomyopathies, skeletal myopathies, ptosis, unusual seizures (e.g., myoclonic epilepsy), diabetes, or optic atrophy. Elevated blood lactate could be the entrance key to this group of disorders, many of which are yielding to the diagnostic tools of the molecular geneticists after years of dependence on muscle biopsy for diagnosis.

The bottom line here: biochemical and molecular testing generally should be left to the discretion of the consultant, although a blood lactate study is a good test to do if a mitochondrial defect comes to mind. It should be noted that rapid progress is being made in identifying and cloning the mutations responsible for specific syndromes.

ARRIVING AT A DIAGNOSIS

By this time you will have a list of findings from your history, physical examination, and laboratory investigations. You scratch your head and think over the list, but still no diagnosis comes to mind. Now what?

Atlas of Malformation Syndromes

If you have an atlas of malformation syndromes available (see Further Reading), you might get lucky. Don't try flipping pages to find a match. Use the tables, usually at the back of the book, listing the common anomalies; many patients will have one or two defects that are more severe or outstanding and you can look for syndromes in which, for example, microphthalmia is often seen. Now you will have a relatively short list of syndromes to match up with your patient. Selection of the defect on which to search is crucial; if you were to choose cleft lip with or without cleft palate, or congenital heart disease, for examples, you would have a list of well over 100 syndromes for each.

The Internet

If you wish to get up-to-date descriptions of even the rarest syndromes, there are several excellent Web sites listed in chapter 1 (Figure 3–33). Unfortunately, at this time, the best of the computer-assisted diagnosis programs (e.g., POSSUM, the London Data Bases) are not on-line but are available in every genetics center. However, Online Mendelian Inheritance in Man (OMIM) is searchable for free and you can do a main anomaly search on that site, often with very helpful results.

Another caveat. No computer or text can examine your patient for you, or take a history. If you don't learn to distinguish abnormal from normal, simple variation from malformation, you're lost!

The Photograph

Be sure to order photographs of your undiagnosed patients: they can be sent to consultants for help with diagnosis and also provide a record of changes that will occur over time. Several syndromes are notoriously difficult to recognize in newborns but may over even a few months become considerably more obvious.

The Consultation

The list of genetics centers for the United States is in the American College of Medical Genetics Guidelines (for Canadian genetics centers, go to the Canadian College of Medical Genetics Web site; for the United Kingdom, see the British Society of Human Genetics; for Europe, the European Society of Human Genetics; and for Australia/New Zealand, the Australasian Human Genetics

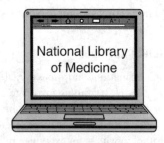

National Library of Medicine

Figure 3–33 Patients should beware of the physician who does not have a computer on his or her desk.

Society) (Figure 3–34). Many of the centers have regularly scheduled outreach clinics and thus, there are few locales where the family will have to travel very far. However, local consultation could be indicated if any of the defects could be life threatening or if a diagnosis is essential before consideration of invasive surgery. For example, referral of a newborn to a distant cardiology service may be contraindicated if the patient has a serious chromosome anomaly or a bone dysplasia syndrome that is uniformly lethal. In addition, having a local colleague look at your puzzling patient could be a big help; two heads are better than one and your colleague just might have seen a similar patient.

MANAGEMENT

Whether or not a specific diagnosis is established, it is essential that the parents and family receive ongoing support. Within the perplexing maze of consultants that so often are necessarily involved, one physician should be primarily concerned with summarizing progress reports, laboratory results, and so on as often as the situation warrants and for providing as upbeat an outlook as possible. The family physician ideally fulfills this role but it could be the family's pediatrician or in the case of a neonate, the neonatologist. There is hardly a situation where *some* sort of treatment won't improve the outlook for the patient; even the most severe congenital cardiac defects can usually be ameliorated, if not totally corrected, by surgery; cleft lips and palates are beautifully reparable; increasing numbers of metabolic diseases can be treated with special diets; missing organs can be transplanted even in infants; and successes with gene therapy will soon outweigh the dismal failures encountered in the closing days of the 20th century. Keep in mind that every couple expects a perfect child and any anomaly is devastating. It might be difficult, after consoling the parents of a severely handicapped child who has trisomy 18, to then turn with equal sympathy to the couple whose infant has isolated polydactyly, but all need your help.

Team management. The child with multiple congenital anomalies will frequently need the expertise of several consultants, sometimes early in a

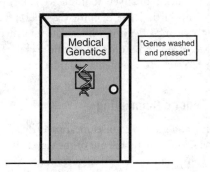

Figure 3–34 The genetics consultation.

pregnancy when anomalies are picked up by fetal ultrasonography. Families find it very helpful to be able to talk directly with a member of, for example, the cardiac surgery team, when a cardiac defect is detected. From the expert they can hear exactly what could be attempted and how likely the procedure is to succeed. When consideration of termination of pregnancy is an issue, these sorts of consultations with the experts are perhaps even more important. As health care turns more routinely to the use of new technology for communication, including computers and two-way TV hookups, families in the more remote communities can be as well counseled as those living near the big centers. Again, the family physician must stay on top of all the consultations and test results so that the family receives consistent input couched in terms they can comprehend.

GENETIC COUNSELING

Although hardly a high priority issue in the early stages of the investigation and management, it will not be very long before the questions arise: Why us? How could this happen when I was so careful during my pregnancy? I never took a drink or a pill, I ate all the right things. Good heavens, if this was genetic, will I ever be able to have a healthy baby? Risks for future offspring and the possibility of prenatal testing or even therapy will need to be discussed when the parents ask the questions, but keep in mind that not very much will be remembered when the child is going through diagnostic studies and therapeutic procedures. In other words, genetic counseling usually requires more than one consultation and again, communication via technology for those in outlying communities is being increasingly successfully used. Even the good old telephone has provided extraordinarily profound relief for many families who have a question that they feel just can't wait for an appointment in 6 weeks or another trip to the medical center. On the other hand, genetic centers are plentiful, as mentioned above.

Following genetic counseling, the family physician still has important roles to fulfill. It is, for example, important to keep in mind that the burden of the condition is much more likely to influence family planning after the birth of a child with a birth defect than the risk figure; for example, a 50% chance of having a second offspring with isolated polydactyly would obviously be much less of a deterrent for having more children than, say, a 1% chance of trisomy 18 with severe mental retardation.

Nondirective Genetic Counseling

Medical geneticists and genetic counselors are acutely aware of the difficulties in keeping one's own prejudices out of the way. Suffice it to say that for the primary-care physician, be careful right from the start to avoid prejudging a family's reaction to even a minor anomaly, never mind a severe one. Let *them* tell *you* how they feel and go from there.

Support Groups

For those patients in whom a specific diagnosis is made, there will be a disease-specific support group to help those families who wish to avail themselves of it, no matter how rare the condition. There is even a National Organization for Rare Diseases (NORD). Virtually all these groups have Web sites and usually provide clear and concise descriptions of the conditions that are relatively free of jargon and available in several languages. Parents and families of, for example, an achondroplastic dwarf, will be virtual fountains of information on the day-to-day issues, such as lowering door handles, judicious placing of step stools, preparation for the inevitable teasing by peers, and the insensitivity of many adults (see chapter 7, "Bone Dysplasias and Short Stature").

An important group is one for couples who have lost a pregnancy through miscarriage, therapeutic abortion, or stillbirth. These families are quite likely to be left to their own devices with a not very reassuring, "You were lucky. The baby would have been so deformed and retarded that it wouldn't have lived anyway." Any of the above types of loss can be shattering and many couples derive a great deal of help and reassurance from others who have had the same experience. The neonatal or obstetrical service will direct couples to an appropriate local pregnancy loss support group. Searching the Internet using **pregnancy loss support groups** plus a local area will usually provide helpful information.

And, as usual, a caveat: The patients whose families seek out support groups tend to be the ones most seriously affected by their condition. You need to discuss that issue with any family thinking about contacting a support group, along with the possibility of the over-exuberant offering of more information and more help than a new family might want all at once.

WEB SITES

"Evaluation of the newborn with single or multiple congenital anomalies: a clinical guideline," is available for downloading from the New York State Department of Health (nysdoh) at <www.health.state.ny.us/nysdoh/dpprd/main.htm#fulldoc>. In it are useful references, tables of measurements, definitions, a list of genetics centers in the US, web sites, and references. Genetics centers for other countries are listed on the sites of their genetics associations: Canadian College of Medical Geneticists, British Society of Human Genetics, European Society of Human Genetics, and Australasian Human Genetics Society.

For **descriptions of syndromes**, often the support group sites (Alliance of Genetic Support Groups, NORD) give the clearest pictures, but sites such as GeneSage and GeneClinics are excellent, if not yet totally complete. OMIM on-line omits little if anything and is gradually being revised so that the clinical descriptions are in separate sections that are easily found rather than being somewhat mixed in among details of the genetics and other issues. To determine whether there is a molecular or biochemical **diagnostic test** for confirmation of diagnosis, GeneTests is an excellent site, although OMIM may continue to have the very latest information since it is so frequently revised and updated.

MEDLINE. I always do a quick check for the very latest information, especially in relation to discovery of the gene responsible for or predisposing to whatever condition I am about to see. It can be embarrassing to have the patient be the first to let you know that the gene for whatever syndrome was cloned and reported or discussed in last month's *JAMA*.

LEARNING POINTS

Problem-Oriented Approach to Birth Defects

Birth defects are common: the incidence at birth is about 1 in 30 and the prevalence at age 7 years is 8% to 9%. A useful classification is as follows:

- Malformations
- Deformations
- Disruptions
- Dysplasias

Solving the diagnostic problem requires a detailed, systematic approach. Why bother?

- Prognosis
- Management and prevention of complications
- Accurate genetic counseling
- Referral to appropriate support group(s)

Physical Examination

The name of the game is to distinguish normal variation from abnormalities and to uncover *all* of the anomalies, both external and internal. Some of the important points to emphasize are:

- First look, don't touch...and look at the patient from different angles.
- Your tape measure—don't leave home without it.
- Physical proportions change with maturation; use tables of measurements, don't trust your memory.

1. **Overandrogenized female**. In other words, a 46,XX biological female exposed to an overabundance of androgens in utero; the usual terminology is a **female pseudohermaphrodite**.
2. **Underandrogenized male**. A 46,XY biological male with insufficient masculinization in utero is referred to as **male pseudohermaphrodite**. As you will recall from embryology, the default system for mammalian sexual development is female; that is, without the turning on of male-determining genes and the intervention of their products, sexual development will proceed as female.
3. **Chromosomal anomaly**. True hermaphroditism and other sex chromosome anomalies, as well as autosomal aneuploidies with ambiguous genitalia as one of a possible constellation of anomalies, fit into this category.
4. **Syndromes with ambiguous genitalia**. Most syndromes with ambiguous genitalia as one of the manifestations are due to single gene mutations; others have multifactorial etiologies.

Now it should be obvious what your next steps should be. Getting to the correct category of diagnoses depends on the karyotype. However, it is imperative to avoid having the baby die of the **one potentially lethal condition**, congenital adrenal hyperplasia, the salt-losing type, while you are waiting for the results of the chromosome analysis or for the consultant to arrive! The diagnostic test result is an increased serum 17-hydroxyprogesterone. In fact, the single most common cause of ambiguous genitalia is congenital adrenal hyperplasia, although not necessarily the salt-losing variety. Let's start with the adrenal cortex and its relationship with abnormal genitalia.

FEMALE PSEUDOHERMAPHRODITISM

1. Congenital Adrenal Hyperplasia Due to P-450c21-hydroxylase Deficiency

The so-called classic form of congenital adrenal hyperplasia (CAH) is the most common cause of female pseudohermaphroditism. Typically, the patient is a chromosomally normal, 46,XX girl who has been masculinized to varying degrees. The vast majority of cases are due to 21-hydroxylase deficiency. Although the inheritance is autosomal recessive, with homozygous males and females affected equally frequently, historically it was believed that it was primarily a disease of females. The excess androgen production in utero masculinizes the female external genitalia to varying degrees but curiously, boys do not present with macropenis at birth, thus delaying the diagnosis as long as the infant is not a salt loser. Affected boys with the salt-losing form of CAH often die misdiagnosed in the neonatal period with clinical features resembling an addisonian crisis—vomiting and diarrhea with severe electrolyte imbalance (low sodium, high potassium), acidosis, and hypovolemia. Hyperpigmentation of the scrotum is a diagnostic clue. All of the clinical manifestations are easily explicable by referring to the diagram of steroid metabolism (Figure 4–2).

Clinical-Biochemical Features

Have a good look at Figure 4–2 and don't panic—it all makes sense. Circle #1 marks the site of the anomaly. *CYP21* is the name of the gene and deficient activity of its product, P-450c21-hydroxylase, or just plain 21-hydroxylase in the older terminology, is responsible for more than 95% of cases of CAH. *CYP21* is in the human leukocyte antigen (HLA) complex on chromosome 6p. This region is known to be a site of frequent recombination and that, presumably, is the explanation, at least in part, for the unusual array of mutational variability in the manifestations of the disease.

About two-thirds of affected patients are salt losers because of the concomitant block in the aldosterone pathway. Why *all* affected individuals aren't salt losers is more of a question; the answer presumably is that some mutations lead to a total absence of 21-hydroxylase activity while others cause a partial lack of the enzyme and hence the range in severity of anomalies.

The normal development of the external genitalia in the male fetus is controlled by androgen, whereas the female requires no exposure to androgens. Girls affected with CAH have excess androgens from their adrenal glands and become masculinized to varying degrees. Some show only mild to moderate clitoromegaly. Others have labioscrotal fusion and a urogenital sinus. Often the labia are "scrotalized" with rugae resembling a bifid scrotum; the infant in Figure 4–1 is an example. Rarely, there is what appears to be a normal penis without hypospadias and bilateral cryptorchidism. The internal female organs develop normally since they are not affected by androgens.

In the salt-losing form, the low levels of aldosterone reduce sodium resorption in the renal tubules, resulting in hypovolemia, hyponatremia, and hyperkalemia. Without treatment, shock and death can occur in the second to third week of life.

The inefficient synthesis of cortisol distal to the block in the pathway leads to a lack of negative feedback to the fetal pituitary gland and this, in turn, causes elevated levels of adrenocorticotropic hormone (ACTH). Hyperpigmentation can result from increased levels of other peptides derived from the ACTH precursor, in particular pro-opiomelanocortin. Pigment distribution is similar to that seen in Addison's disease with brown discoloration in the creases of the extremities, the labioscrotal folds, and clitoris. The overproduction of ACTH also results in oversynthesis of androstenedione ($\Delta4$), which is converted to excess amounts of the potent androgen testosterone; hence the masculinization of the genetic female.

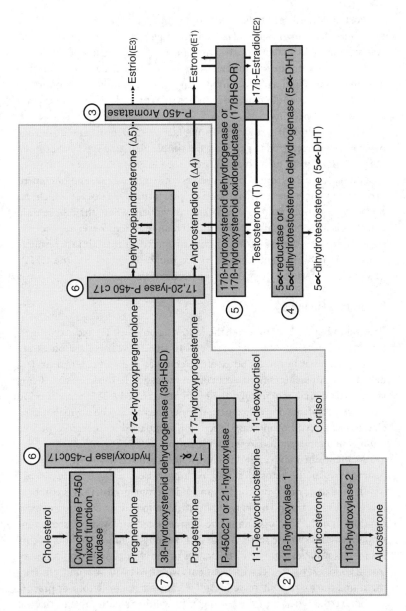

Figure 4–2 The biosynthesis of steroids. The metabolic pathways within the shaded box exist within the adrenal cortex. Those outside the box take place in the fetal gonad, the placenta, and other tissues. The circled numbers refer to the disorders discussed in the text.

Postnatally, untreated girls and boys with mild or no salt loss will have rapid somatic growth with advanced bone age, premature closure of the epiphyses, and ultimately, short stature. Boys develop a macropenis usually by 2 to 3 years of age and undergo premature sexual development with growth of pubic and axillary hair and appearance of adult body odor; the testes remain prepubertal since the premature development is not gonadotropin mediated.

The one-third of patients with normal or near-normal aldosterone biosynthesis are referred to as having the **simple virilizing** type. In addition, there is a **nonclassic** form, typically expressed in girls at puberty with manifestations resulting from androgen excess: hirsutism, acne, and oligomenorrhea or amenorrhea. There is even a **cryptic** form of the disease, which was uncovered in family studies of affected individuals, where the biochemical defect(s) is present but detectable clinical manifestations never appear.

In summary, there is a broad clinical spectrum that almost certainly reflects the heterogeneous nature of the mutations involving the *CYP21* gene and its effects on 21-hydroxylase production.

Laboratory Findings

Referral to Figure 4–2 will make the following obvious: 17-hydroxyprogesterone and other precursors proximal to the 21-hydroxylase block are greatly increased in the blood in all three types of P-450c21-hydroxylase deficiency (salt losing, simple virilizing, nonclassic). In the simple virilizing type, cortisol is close to normal as a result of increased ACTH secretion and a relatively mild enzyme deficiency. Aldosterone can also be normal or even elevated as a result of increased secretion stimulated by increased plasma renin activity in response to the salt loss.

As mentioned above, the diagnostic test is for serum 17-hydroxyprogesterone; urine 17-ketosteroids are no longer used.

In the salt-losing type, cortisol and aldosterone production is compromised. ACTH cannot compensate by stimulating sufficient cortisol production, and the salt loss cannot be compensated for by increased renin-stimulated aldosterone secretion. In fact, a rising serum renin level occurs before either the electrolyte disturbances or the clinical signs and is, therefore, a good test to predict which patients with CAH will be salt losers. Furthermore, the marked increase in ACTH causes a major detour of precursors above the block into the androgen biosynthesis pathway and that, of course, worsens the androgen effects on the external genitalia.

Management

There are five important issues that require your attention and that need to be discussed with patients' parents. See how many you can come up with before reading on.

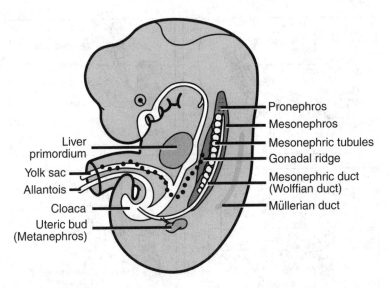

Figure 4–3 The structure of the embryonic urogenital system at 5 weeks. The black dots represent the migrating primordial germ cells from the yolk sac into the gonad ridge via the allantois and the developing hindgut (not shown).

are composed of somatic mesodermal cells plus primordial germ cells that have formed at the base of the allantois and migrated to the genital ridges via the hindgut and mesonephros (see Figure 4–3).

The primordial germ cells arise in the yolk sac starting at the 4th week and migrate, as mentioned above, to enter the gonadal ridge at the 6th week, where they are incorporated into the primary sex cords.

Male Sex Differentiation

Testicular differentiation is evident by 7 weeks gestation. By 8 weeks, the germ cells number about 500,000 and the primitive sex cords (also known as the seminiferous or testicular cords) have grown into the intermediate mesoderm. This mesenchyme gives rise to Leydig's or interstitial cells between the 8th and 9th weeks. At about the same time, Sertoli's cells develop from the primitive sex cords. Their specific products and their roles in sex differentiation are summarized in Figure 4–5 and Figure 4–6. It will help you to keep the events straight if you refer to those figures from time to time.

Sertoli's cell differentiation may be *triggered* by *SRY*, with expression *regulated* by *SF1* (steroidogenic factor-1). The Sertoli's cells produce a number of products (see Figure 4–5), most prominently müllerian-inhibiting substance (MIS), also known as müllerian-inhibiting factor or antimüllerian hormone

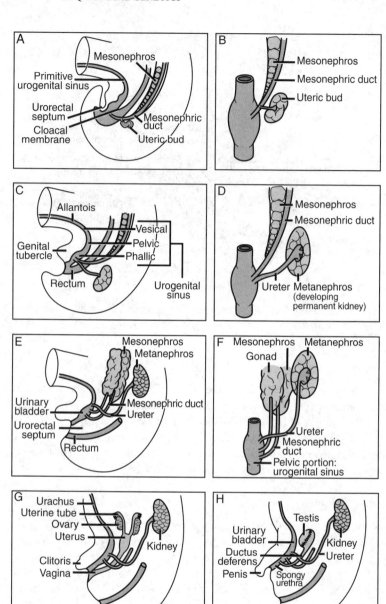

Figure 4–4 These diagrams depict the early stages of human embryonic development (5th–12th weeks) at the caudal end. Lateral views are on the left; dorsal on the right. *A* and *B*, represent a 5-week-old embryo and from *A* to *F*, there is no visible sex differentiation. The stages reached in *G* and *H* are at the 12th week. The factors controlling the stages of development up to the time of secretion of testosterone by the testes at about 7 weeks are not yet known. (From Moore and Persaud, 1998)

ensure that the ovaries do not; that is, there is sexual dimorphism in steroid biosynthesis in the embryo.

III. Gender Identification and Sexual Behavior

The Flea

Here's the happy bounding flea—
You cannot tell the he from she.
The sexes look alike, you see;
But she can tell, and so can he.

Roland Young, c1950

The plethora of genes influencing sex determination already identified and discussed above should make it abundantly clear that gender identification is extremely complex. Mutations that lead to a variety of aberrant sexual behaviors have been detected and mapped in *Drosophila*, and there is no question that many of the sex hormones that are synthesized early in the embryo have effects on parts of the body other than the sex organs, including, most importantly, the brain. The belief that the sex of a child can be reversed without harm up to 18 months of age, as proposed by Money and his colleagues decades ago, has been vigorously challenged in recent years. Support groups are willing and able assistants in providing information for both physicians and patients; the two most influential ones are the Androgen Insensitivity Syndrome (AIS) support group with branches in the United Kingdom, North America, and Australia, and the Intersex Society of North America (ISNA). The Web site address for the latter and a link to the former are included among the references at the end of the chapter.

The nature–nurture debate on the etiology of homosexuality literally rages in the pages of both scientific journals and the public press. What is clear is that there is no gene *for* homosexual orientation any more than there is a gene *for* heterosexual orientation. Suffice it to say for these pages that sexual identification is a complex trait in humans and, for that matter, among most living organisms, and the nature of the interactions among the genome, development, and life experiences has yet to be worked out.

MALE PSEUDOHERMAPHRODITISM

We're now talking about the 46,XY male who is underandrogenized and therefore has varying degrees of genital ambiguity. There are only two etiological possibilities: underproduction of androgen or a defect in androgen action at the target tissues.

1. Underproduction of Androgen

5α-Dehydrotestosterone Dehydrogenase Deficiency

Also called 5α-reductase, type 2, deficiency (see Figure 4–2, circle #4), this is by far the most common of the group of *hormonal* causes of male pseudo-hermaphroditism. The enzyme, existing as two isozymes, converts testosterone to its more potent form, 5α-DHT. Type 1 5α-DHT dehydrogenase is not expressed in utero. The inheritance of type 2 deficiency is autosomal recessive and clinically, most affected boys appear female at birth; some, however, have ambiguous genitalia with a small hypospadic phallus, bifid scrotum, hypoplastic prostate, and a blind vaginal pouch with a single urethral and vaginal opening (urogenital sinus). The testes are nearly always extra-abdominal, lying in the inguinal canal or scrotum.

Diagnosis. Testosterone levels should be normal but the testosterone-to-DHT ratio is increased. The normal ratio is 5:10; it can exceed 20 in 5α-DHT-deficient subjects. Direct assay of 5α-reductase also can be done on cultured genital skin fibroblasts.

Management. Management will depend on the degree of genital anomaly and the outcome of counseling the parents. Daily application of 5α-DHT cream to the penis and genital areas should increase penis size. Surgery might be indicated, depending on the selected sex of rearing, and prepubertal hormone therapy might increase muscle bulk, hair growth, and libido.

17β-Hydroxysteroid Dehydrogenase Deficiency

The site of the block is shown in Figure 4–2 and designated as circle #5. There are several isozymes of 17β-hydroxysteroid dehydrogenase (17β-HSD), each encoded by different autosomal genes. Mutations in isozyme type 3, responsible for conversion of androstenedione ($\Delta 4$) to testosterone (T), as in Figure 4–2, are the most common causes of undervirilization due to defective testosterone synthesis but are nevertheless rare. Inheritance is autosomal recessive and the clinical manifestations are similar to those described above for 5α-DHT deficiency—most appear female; some have ambiguity. Those with apparent female external genitalia will often have a blind vagina with either inguinal hernia or "labial" masses. Internal structures include the epididymis, vas deferens, seminal vesicles, and ejaculatory duct; that is, the wolffian duct derivatives. The pathogenesis raises many questions regarding the precise roles of the sex steroid in development of the various parts of the anatomy; for example, why are there internal wolffian duct derivatives and female external genitalia, and why does breast development occur at puberty? The latter could result from conversion of E_1 to E_2.

Diagnosis. Plasma Δ4 and estrone are elevated; testosterone and estradiol (E_2) are relatively low.

Management. Management is as above for DHT deficiency. Those patients raised as girls will show marked virilization at puberty with clitoral enlargement, increased muscle mass, and masculine-appearing physique. The issues of gender will have to be addressed with care at that time.

P-450c17 Deficiency

P-450c17 is a bifunctional enzyme responsible for 17α-hydroxylase and 17,20-lyase activities (see Figure 4–2, circle #6). Deficiencies of androgen, estrogen, and cortisol occur but in some patients there is an increase of mineralocorticoids. The condition is very rare and as with the above two, external genitalia are variable, sometimes ambiguous. Overproduction of mineralocorticoids can cause hypertension and hypokalemia. The 46,XY individuals have a female phenotype and no sex steroid production in puberty. They have no uterus and thus, do not menstruate at puberty, even with estrogen therapy, although breast growth is good. The 46,XX individuals do not develop breasts and do develop hypertension. They will mature with estrogen treatment and will menstruate but are infertile.

    Diagnosis. Elevated levels of the precursors pregnenolone and progesterone and deficiencies of their products, as is evident in the pathways of Figure 4–2, indicate the condition.

3β-Hydroxysteroid Dehydrogenase Deficiency

Another rare autosomal recessive cause of CAH (circle #7 in Figure 4–2), with undermasculinization and with or without salt loss, is 3β-hydroxysteroid dehydrogenase (3β-HSD) deficiency. The diagnosis is made by finding an elevated Δ5/Δ4 ratio. However, plasma steroid profiles can be confusing and direct molecular sequencing of amplified DNA fragments from the 3β-HSD gene might be required.

2. Defects in Androgen Action at the Target Tissues (Androgen Insenstivity Syndromes)

Androgen receptor (AR) is a nuclear receptor protein that binds androgen. It is encoded by a gene on the short arm of the X chromosome (Xq11-12). The androgen-AR complex becomes a transcription factor that dimerizes and binds to certain regulatory sequences of DNA to regulate expression of androgen target genes controlled by nearby promoters. Defects in AR cause male pseudohermaphroditism.

    A sufficient amount of structurally normal AR must be available at specific times during development so that androgens can control (i.e., switch on or off) expression of genes whose products effect normal masculinization of a male embryo, as well as effect normal virilization at puberty.

Estrogen receptor (ER) defects cause a very rare autosomal recessive disorder that is believed to be almost always embryologically lethal, possibly because it impairs placental implantation. The rare humans detected with the condition have not had ambiguous genitalia.

Clinically, there are three classes of androgen insensitivity severity:

1. **Total androgen insensitivity**. The first class is total androgen insensitivity or "testicular feminization" as it was inappropriately called in the past. The phenotype is a normal or near-normal female at birth, although inguinal herniation of one or both testes is not uncommon. The vagina is usually a blind pouch and the uterus is absent or vestigial. At puberty, breast development occurs with absent pubic and axillary hair and, of course, no menarche. The diagnosis for the first affected person in a family is usually made in the teens.
2. **Partial androgen insensitivity**. As one would expect, there are highly variable degrees of ambiguity of the external and internal genitalia.
3. **Mild androgen insensitivity**. Genital structures are normal or near normal. Affected males may have generalized microgenitalia—small penis and small scrotum; occasionally mild hypospadias. Testes usually are descended and of normal size.

Diagnosis

Testosterone and 5α-DHT are normal or elevated, and there is a normal testosterone/DHT ratio. A definitive diagnosis can be established by direct assay of AR activity in cultured genital skin fibroblasts.

Management

Patients with total androgen insensitivity are almost invariably well-adjusted girls by the time the diagnosis is made. Obviously, testes should be removed and the patient and family appropriately counseled by an experienced team. For patients with ambiguous genitalia due to partial androgen sensitivity, sensitive counseling is indicated with subsequent attempts to promote male sex development by androgen therapy. Surgery might be beneficial when the sex of rearing is clearly established.

CHROMOSOME ANOMALIES

True Hermaphroditism

A hermaphrodite, by definition, is an organism in which reproductive organs of both sexes are present. In humans, that implies both ovarian and testicular tissue, most often, but not necessarily, as an ovotestis. Some prefer the euphemism **intersex** rather than the term hermaphrodite.

According to Greek mythology, Hermaphrodite, or Hermaphroditus, was the son of Hermes (Mercury, for the Romans) who, among other things, was the messenger for his father, Zeus. Hermes wore a winged cap and winged shoes and carried a rod entwined with two serpents, the caduceus, which became the symbol of the medical profession. Its resemblance to the double helix of DNA is appropriate and prophetic, now that genetics has become the focal point for all of medicine! Aphrodite, also known as Venus, the goddess of love, was Hermaphroditus's mother. Legend has it that a nymph, upon seeing the young Hermaphroditus bathing in a fountain, fell hopelessly in love with him. She begged the gods to let their bodies become one and through this myth, the Greeks projected the physical ideals of both male and female onto the figure of Hermaphroditus.

The karyotype runs the gamut from 46,XY to 46,XX and a variety of sex chromosome mosaics. Curiously, 46,XX is by far the most common karyotype and there are both familial and sporadic types. Although it was suspected that Y chromosomal sequences were translocated to somewhere in the 46,XX hermaphrodite, at least in the familial forms, searches have yielded negative results even with sensitive new techniques for detection of Y chromosomal material and *SRY* transcripts.

Clinically, the condition is detected at birth because of the ambiguous genitalia. Other congenital anomalies are rare. Occasionally, instead of an ovotestis, some patients have a testis on one side, usually the right, and an ovary on the left. The other internal genital organs are highly variable but always include at least remnants of both müllerian and wolffian structures.

Diagnosis usually can be established through imaging studies and laparoscopy. Plasma testosterone levels can be high for 46,XX females and hCG-stimulated testosterone values will indicate the presence of testicular tissue. In the 46,XX individuals, no specific mutations have been identified in any gene and, as mentioned above, *SRY* and other Y chromosomal sequences are not found. Of interest is the fact that several XX hermaphrodites have had anomalies of chromosome 22, most often duplications, but occasionally partial and even complete trisomy. 46,XX true hermaphrodites are fertile if they have an ovary that is distinct from the testes or ovotestis. In contrast, the testes fail to make sperm and these males are infertile.

XX/XY Mosaic True Hermaphroditism

Although a rare cause of genital ambiguity, this condition merits a brief mention because of the issue of striking ascertainment bias. Postnatal ascertainment occurs because a karyotype is done during the course of an evaluation of ambiguous genitalia. However, if an XX/XY mosaic is detected in a fetus on amniocentesis, the vast majority will turn out to be phenotypically normal males. Nevertheless, before providing too optimistic a prognosis for the prenatally detected cases, the fetus should be carefully examined by level II ultrasonography, focused particularly on genital structures and kidneys (renal dysgenesis and aplasia are sometimes associated with the condition).

Another point worth emphasis is the fact that the presence of a dysgenetic gonad of any type in association with any Y chromosome mosaicism puts the individual at increased risk of gonadoblastoma and the dysplastic gonad must be removed. The risk of tumor is small before puberty but there have been a few childhood cases reported and the gonad should be removed when the karyotype is determined.

Most other chromosome anomalies involving either the X or Y chromosome are not associated with ambiguous genitalia.

Autosomal Aneuploidy

Almost invariably, the external genital anomaly is seen in association with other congenital anomalies and actual ambiguity is far less common than the various forms of hypoplasia, including cryptorchidism, chordee, and hypospadias in males, and labial fusion or hypoplasia of the labia in females. The message, as emphasized in chapter 3, "Approach to the Child With Congenital Malformations," is the importance of developing a systematic approach that includes a careful history, examination of the patient as well as the parents, and of course, a karyotype, among other laboratory studies, as indicated.

SYNDROMES WITH AMBIGUOUS GENITALIA AS ONE MANIFESTATION

Using OMIM, searching for "ambiguous genitalia" yielded 43 entries, many of which have already been mentioned. (The numbers in parentheses are the OMIM numbers.) These include the *WT1* locus (194070), the various types of congenital adrenal hyperplasia, the androgen insensitivity syndromes (313700), and true hermaphroditism (235600). The rest are rare conditions, most inherited as autosomal recessive traits. Again, the approach to diagnosis is as described in chapter 3. At this time, perhaps one condition bears mentioning.

Smith-Lemli-Opitz Syndrome

Smith-Lemli-Opitz syndrome (SLOS; 270400) merits a note for several reasons. It is caused by an inherited defect of cholesterol synthesis and the incidence is currently estimated at between 1:20,000 and 1:40,000, making it the second most common autosomal recessive condition causing mental retardation after phenylketonuria. Now that there is a relatively simple diagnostic test for the disorder, the variability will emerge and it could turn out to be even more prevalent. The defect, an enzymatic deficiency of 3β-hydroxysteroid Δ7 reductase due to mutations of the reductase gene, *DHCR7*, leads to a generalized deficiency of cholesterol and accumulation of its precursors, 7-dehydrocholesterol (DHC) and 8-DHC, in body fluids.

Clinically, the most striking features are postaxial polydactyly, syndactyly of the 2nd and 3rd toes, often complete, and external anomalies of the genitalia. In addition, there is dysmorphism (microcephaly or holoprosencephaly, micrognathia, blepharoptosis, flat nasal bridge, anteverted nares, cleft palate, and congenital cataracts). The typical overlapping of the index finger, as seen in trisomy 18, occurs fairly frequently, and there are often severe anomalies of the heart, great vessels, gastrointestinal tract, genitourinary tract, and brain. Failure to thrive, both intrauterine and postnatal, is almost invariable. I often think of SLOS when I've initially suspected trisomy 18 and the karyotype comes back as normal.

The diagnosis depends on laboratory determination of an elevated 7-DHC in the blood, usually in association with low levels of cholesterol. Prenatal diagnosis can be made through amniotic fluid analysis of 7-DHC and cholesterol. However, DNA testing is being used with increasing frequency. It should be noted that on the maternal serum screen many cases of SLOS will test positive for Down syndrome or trisomy 18 due to impaired estriol synthesis. The prenatal presentation, in addition to detection of the anomalies above, can include nuchal edema with or without fetal hydrops, probably due to fetal heart failure secondary to an anatomical defect.

Management by oral supplementation of cholesterol is under investigation. Growth and behavior improve but whether there will be significant improvement in intellectual development remains to be seen.

Clinical Scenario: The Denouement

Let's return to the clinical scenario. The serum level of 17-hydroxy-progesterone was markedly elevated and the serum electrolytes were normal and remained so. A renin assay was done to detect the possibility of a compensated salt loser, and it was normal. The karyotype was 46,XX and thus, the infant was diagnosed as having CAH due to P-450c21 or 21-hydroxylase deficiency, the simple virilizing type. The external genitalia were as shown in Figure 4–1, and there was a urogenital sinus. Treatment with cortisol was initiated as soon as the diagnosis was established in order to stop any further masculinization.

The parents were, of course, deeply concerned about the operations looming for the future and in the course of the consultations inquired about the outlook for future children. The one-in-four risk of another affected child was explained and the concern, of course, would be another affected girl; there would be a one-in-eight chance of that happening. Prenatal diagnosis of an affected fetus and identification of fetal sex would not be difficult, but the couple was very hesitant regarding termination of pregnancy for a treatable disorder with no risk of intellectual impairment. Fortunately, as explained by the geneticist who was called in for consultation, CAH represents the first genetic condition that has been successfully treated medically while the fetus is in utero. The following approach was outlined for all future pregnancies:

- *As soon as pregnancy is confirmed, the mother would be started on a glucocorticoid (dexamethasone) to suppress the fetal pituitary in case an affected female had been conceived. It is essential to start therapy as soon as possible since testosterone synthesis commences at 7 to 8 weeks' gestation.*
- *The parents could choose chorionic villus sampling or amniocentesis to establish the sex of the fetus and to determine whether or not it is affected.*
- *Maternal treatment can be stopped for a male fetus or an unaffected female.*
- *If the fetus is determined to be an affected female, maternal dexamethasone should be continued throughout the pregnancy.*

Several studies have shown that as long as maternal therapy is started at between 5 and 9 weeks with adequate dosage, the majority of affected girls are born with normal or only mildly masculinized external genitalia. To date, documented maternal side effects have included excess weight gain, hypertension, increased urinary glucose, and striae; many women report being quite miserable during the treatment period with insomnia and mood swings, in addition to various combinations of the above.

LEARNING POINTS

The four etiological categories for ambiguous genitalia are as follows:

1. Masculinization of a 46,XX female (female pseudohermaphroditism)
2. Undermasculinization of a 46,XY male (male pseudohermaphroditism)
3. Chromosome disorder (true hermaphroditism and others)
4. Syndrome with ambiguous genitalia as one of a constellation of anomalies

The specific disorders for each etiological category are as follows:

1. Female pseudohermaphroditism
   - Congenital adrenal hyperplasia (CAH) due to P-450c21-hydroxylase deficiency
   - CAH due to 11β-hydroxylase deficiency
   - Aromatase deficiency

- Virilizing maternal tumors
- Exogenous androgen
- Fetal tumors with infiltration of external genitalia
2. Male pseudohermaphroditism
   - Underproduction of androgen due to 5α-DHT dehydrogenase (5α-reductase) deficiency, 17β-HSD deficiency, P-450c17 deficiency, or 3β-HSD deficiency
   - Abnormal androgen action (partial androgen receptor defects)
3. Chromosomal anomalies (true hermaphroditism, sex chromosome mosaicism, autosomal aneuploidy)
4. Syndromes (e.g., Smith-Lemli-Opitz syndrome)

Warning: Avoid having the infant die of salt loss while you're sorting out the diagnosis! The danger period is the second to third week of life.

Mammalian Sex Determination

Embryology

1. Indifferent stage
   - Anatomy of sexual development is identical in the sexes until about the 5th week of gestation
   - Urogenital system develops in the caudal portion of the embryo from the intermediate mesoderm; the wolffian and müllerian duct systems appear
   - Without the action of *SRY*, the müllerian ducts form the uterus, oviducts, and upper vagina
   - Gonads and genital ridges arise from the mesonephros
   - Primordial germ cells arise in the yolk sac and migrate to enter the gonadal ridge at the 6th week
2. Male sex differentiation
   - Testis differentiation evident by 7 weeks
   - Sertoli's cells → AMH by the 8th week plus AMH receptor molecules
   - Leydig's cells → testosterone at about 9 weeks, which, via the AR receptor molecules, directs development of the wolffian ducts toward ejaculatory ducts, vas deferens, seminal vesicles, and epididymis
3. Female sex differentiation
   - The default system!
   - However, sufficient aromatase activity must be present to convert androgens from the fetal adrenal to estrogens
   - At approximately 12 weeks, germ cells proliferate and become recognizable as oogonia and then oocytes

- By 16 weeks, follicle production begins; surviving oocytes are arrested in prophase of meiosis I
4. External genitalia development
   - By the 4th week the genital tubercle is forming similarly in both sexes
   - By the 6th week, the cloaca has a urogenital sinus anteriorly and the rectum and anus posteriorly
   - DHT is the determining factor for differentiation of the external male genitalia

Molecular and Biochemical Aspects of Sex Differentiation

- Prior to the expression of *SRY*, three genes implicated in gonadal development are functioning: *SF1*, *WT1*, and *LIM1*
- *SRY* is the TDF gene; its target cells and the genes that it regulates are still not totally understood. Candidates include Sertoli's cells, *SOX9*, and *SF1*.
- *DAX1*, the gene responsible for adrenal hypoplasia congenita, is X-linked and plays a poorly understood role in sex differentiation
- Autosomal genes: *SOX9*, *WT1*, *SF1*, and *DMRT1*. All are involved in ways that have yet to be clarified
- *GATA4*, another autosomal gene, is involved in regulation of AMH, along with *SOX9*, *SF1*, and *WT1*.
- INSL3 is required for descent of the testes

Gender Identification

Gender identification is the result of a complex interaction of developmental genes, intrauterine environment, and life experiences.

References

1. Shozu M, Akasofu K, Harada T, Kubota Y. A new cause of female pseudohermaphroditism: placental aromatase deficiency. J Clin Endocrinol Metab 1991;72:560–6.

Further Reading

Congenital Adrenal Hyperplasia and Ambiguous Genitalia

Carlson AD, Obeid JS, Kanellopoulou N, et al. Congenital adrenal hyperplasia: update on prenatal diagnosis and treatment. J Steroid Biochem Mol Biol 1999; 69:19–29.
Pang S. Congenital adrenal hyperplasia. Baillieres Clin Obstet Gynaecol 1997;11: 281–306.

Pinsky L, Erickson RP, Schimke RN. Genetic disorders of human sexual development. New York: Oxford University Press; 1999.

Mammalian Sex Determination

Hines M. Abnormal sexual development and psychosexual issues. Baillieres Clin Endocrinol Metab 1998;12:173–89.

Money J, Hampson JC, Hampson JL. Hermaphroditism: recommendations concerning assignment of sex, and psychologic management. Johns Hopkins Med J 1955;97:284–95.

Moore KL, Persaud TVN. The developing human: clinically oriented embryology. 6th ed. Philadelphia: WB Saunders; 1998.

Roberts LM, Shen J, Ingraham HA. Human genetics '99: sexual development. New solutions to an ancient riddle: defining the differences between Adam and Eve. Am J Hum Genet 1999;65:933–42.

Schafer AJ. Sex determination and its pathology in man. Adv Genet 1995;33:275–329.

Swain A, Lovell-Badge R. Mammalian sex determination: a molecular drama. Genes Dev 1999;13:755–67.

Androgen Insensitivity Syndromes

Ahmed SF, Hughes IA. The genetics of male undermasculinization. Clin Endocrinol 2002;56:1–18.

Gottleib B, Pinsky L, Beitel LK, et al. Androgen insensitivity. Am J Med Genet 1999;89:210–17.

Web Sites

Androgen Insensitivity Syndrome Support Group   <www.medhelp.org/www/ais>
Intersex Society of North America   <www.isna.org>

Newborn Screening

Genetic screening can be defined as a search in a population for persons possessing certain genotypes that (1) are already associated with disease or predispose to disease, (2) could lead to disease in their descendants, or (3) produce other variations not known to be associated with disease. Persons in the first category are identified so that medical management can be provided, the second group is discovered so that reproductive options can be discussed, and the third category gathers information for research purposes—that is, for the study of the genetic constitutions of populations. This chapter deals with category 1 and chapter 6, "Pregnancy and Prepregnancy Genetic Screening," deals with category 2.

Newborn genetic screening can be defined as a search for asymptomatic newborn infants who have inherited a disease that through early diagnosis and institution of medical management will have its manifestations either prevented or greatly minimized.

PHENYLKETONURIA

Clinical Scenario

You receive a phone call from the regional laboratory right at the end of the day: your first positive phenylketonuria (PKU) test on a baby you delivered a few days ago. It had been a perfect first pregnancy for the Smiths with an uncomplicated labor and delivery. Melanie had let the world know she'd arrived with a lusty cry, and she was eating and sleeping just as she was supposed to do. You figured it would be best to stop by the Smith home to give them the bad news on your way home; it's on your way and would save you trying to squeeze them into a crowded office schedule. In addition, it would give you time to explain the whole thing to them before referring them to the metabolic unit at the regional health center. You're almost certain that they won't even remember that there was a test pending on the baby . . . and you were right!

Melanie was exactly 1 week old. Bob and Sal Smith were having a little birthday celebration—a martini for the proud Dad and just a sip of wine for Mom; she was breastfeeding. Now you had to tell them that a test done on a drop of blood taken from the baby's heel shortly after delivery showed that most likely she had an inherited condition called phenylketonuria and that although it is potentially serious, preventive treatment is available and most babies with PKU develop normally in every way. Needless to say, tears and questions flowed. You gave them some introductory information while assuring them that the metabolic program would have all the details and would help them with Melanie's care literally throughout her childhood and into adolescence. One thing that initially confused them more than anything else was the hereditary part. Both Bob and Sal came from fairly large families; most of the relatives, including the grandparents, lived to ripe old ages. There was no history of any unusual diseases, no one was mentally handicapped and certainly no babies got sick or needed special diets.

The issues raised in this clinical scenario are:

- What is newborn screening?
- What conditions are currently screened for in most North American and European countries?
- Why don't we screen for more genetic diseases?
- How common are the conditions we do screen for?
- Does a positive test for PKU mean that the child has the disease?
- What about false negatives?
- What are the risks for future pregnancies?
- What can we anticipate for the future in newborn screening?

Before dealing with these questions, let's have a quick look at this disease, PKU. Although it is quite rare, with incidences from one in 10,000 to one in 15,000 live births in various populations, it is, nevertheless, one of the most common of the inborn errors of metabolism and, like most, is inherited as an autosomal recessive trait. Prior to initiation of newborn screening using filter-paper blood spots in the 1960s, PKU accounted for 0.5% to 1% of patients in institutions for the mentally retarded. It is due to deficient activity of the enzyme phenylalanine hydroxylase, which processes the amino acid phenylalanine, and the block in metabolism leads to increased amounts of phenylalanine in the blood and other tissues. Increased amounts of the breakdown products of that amino acid contribute to damage of the developing nervous system, resulting in mental retardation, seizures, and behavioral disorders, as does the deficiency of metabolites, including neurotransmitters distal to the block. The lack of pigmentation of the skin and the irides is due to deficient production of melanin (tyrosinase, the enzyme responsible for the conversion of tyrosine to melanin, is inhibited by excess amounts of phenylalanine). The peculiar musty odor of the untreated patient with PKU is due to accumulating phenylacetic acid. The various steps in the metabolism of phenylalanine are illustrated in Figure 5–1, including the involvement of the tetrahydrobiopterin cofactor, BH4, required for activation of phenylalanine hydroxylase. The same cofactor system is required for the hydroxylation of tyrosine to levodopa in the synthesis of the neurotransmitters paminine, noradrenaline, and adrenaline. Some 5% of infants with hyperphenylalaninemia have defects in the synthesis of BH4 or the activation of dihydropteridine (qBH2) to biopterin. These rare forms of PKU do not respond to dietary therapy alone.

History

In the early 1930s, Dr. I. Asbjorn Folling of Norway was studying children with mental retardation when he discovered a group of them whose urine turned green in the presence of ferric chloride. Folling identified excess amounts of phenylpyruvic acid as the cause of the positive ferric chloride test. Three years later, Penrose and Quastel[1] suggested the name phenylketonuria, and it has remained in common use ever since. This ferric chloride urine test worked for confirming the diagnosis of PKU, but it was of no use for the early detection or prevention of the disease because not enough phenylalanine builds up in the early weeks of life to cause its metabolites to appear in sufficient amounts in the urine for a positive test. Therefore detection would be too late for the institution of treatment to prevent damage. The possibility of treating or preventing the disease was, of course, unknown to these early investigators.

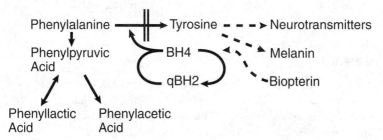

Figure 5–1 Metabolism of phenylalanine, including the biopterin cofactor system. The block due to deficient phenylalanine hydroxylase activity is indicated by the double vertical lines.

In 1939, a physician, George A. Jervis, demonstrated that PKU is hereditary and showed that there were increased amounts of phenylalanine and its metabolites in the blood and other tissues, as well as in the urine. But it wasn't until 1953 that a German physician, Horst Bickel, working with colleagues in England, developed the low-phenylalanine diet for the treatment of PKU.

The test in current use, which is responsible for the launching of newborn screening for genetic disorders, was developed by Robert Guthrie, MD, PhD (microbiology)—only a physician with a background of work with microorganisms would be likely to come up with the following approach. He and his colleagues had found that growth in culture of the microorganism *Bacillus subtilis* was inhibited by β-2-thienylalanine, an analogue of phenylalanine, in the medium. This inhibition could be overcome by the addition to the culture medium of several metabolites, including phenylalanine and phenylpyruvic acid. Thus, Guthrie was able to develop a convenient agar diffusion microbial assay employing small filter-paper discs impregnated with blood serum on the agar surface. The test was calibrated and perfected on patients being treated. The system is very neat: phenylalanine in the blood diffuses out into the agar during an overnight incubation of the plate. The *B. subtilis* inhibition is overcome and a ring of bacterial growth appears around any blood spots with increased amounts of phenylalanine. Discs from normal infants showed almost undetectable surrounding rings of growth. The size of the ring of bacterial growth is in direct proportion to the amount of phenylalanine in the blood spot. Each plate is calibrated for semiquantitative assay using filter-paper spots with known amounts of phenylalanine, as shown in Figure 5–2.

This simple but ingenious technique initiated the concept of newborn screening for the diagnosis and prevention of mental handicap due to inherited metabolic diseases.[2] Technology to automate the punching out of highly uniform filter-paper discs was developed along with procedures to detect additional metabolic diseases, hemoglobinopathies (e.g., sickle cell disease), thyroid hormone deficiency (cretinism), and immunological conditions.

Genetics

There is more to the genetic aspects than meets the eye! PKU is believed by most medical practitioners to be an autosomal recessive inherited disease wherein affected individuals are homozygous for identical mutant alleles and where there is a clear distinction between affected and normal individuals. However, PKU has turned out to be a **complex disorder** (see chapter 2, "Complex Genetic Disorders") even though it is, in essence, an autosomal recessive condition. The first sign of heterogeneity was the discovery, clini-

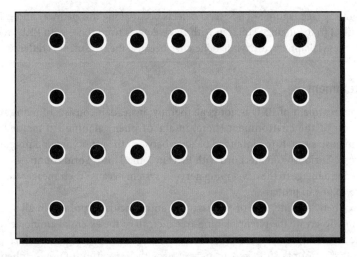

Figure 5–2 Depiction of a typical Guthrie agar diffusion gel. The black dots represent filter-paper blood spots and the white rings, areas of bacterial growth. The top line shows spots impregnated with increasing amounts of phenylalanine from left to right. The third sample in the third row represents a positive Guthrie test from an infant with an elevated blood phenylalanine level.

cally, of non-PKU mild hyperphenylalaninemia (levels of phenylalanine are increased beyond the upper range of normal but no clinical manifestations of PKU ever appear) and a condition now called mild PKU; both are associated with decreased phenylalanine hydroxylase activities. In addition, there is a transient, totally benign, hyperphenylalaninemia of the newborn, seen most frequently in premature infants, unassociated with any of the known mutations, and probably resulting from immaturity of liver enzymes. Patients with classic PKU have virtually absent phenylalanine hydroxylase activity.

The gene for phenylalanine hydroxylase has been cloned and mapped to chromosome 12q24.1. More than 400 mutations have been found so far and the genotypes and biochemical phenotypes are closely related:

- Null mutations are associated with classic PKU.
- Other mutations are associated with mild PKU or mild hyperphenyl-alaninemia.
- Some variability in the biochemical and clinical phenotypes has been obtained for a number of the mutations.

To finish off the story of variability for PKU, between 1% and 5% of infants identified in newborn PKU screening programs have secondary hyper-phenylalaninemia due to a defect in the tetrahydrobiopterin (BH4) cofactor pathway (see Figure 5–1). Several defects occur along this pathway and it is critical to distinguish children with these defects from those with PKU due to phenylalanine hydroxylase deficiency because the treatment is different.

Treatment

The treatment of PKU is not gene therapy; instead, it consists of manipulation of the environment (here, intake of phenylalanine) to maintain homeostasis, nature's intended balance between the genotypes and phenotypes. Curiously, infants born with PKU in some Third World countries can escape damage to the developing nervous system because their meager diets are so low in protein.

Phenylalanine, one of the essential amino acids, is present in all proteins. To create the phenylalanine-free diet, all of the essential amino acids are removed from the infant milk formula and then put back in with controlled amounts sufficient to permit growth but without enough phenylalanine to cause damage to the developing nervous system. This serves as the primary source of protein; other foods such as fruits, vegetables, and cereals, in measured amounts, are also given. It soon became obvious that the diet must be started early, ideally within the first few weeks of life, to be effective in preventing mental retardation. It has to be continued for at least the first 10 years, if not throughout the lifespan of the affected individual, especially for females (see "Maternal PKU" below).

The rare forms of PKU due to cofactor deficiency require inclusion of BH4 and neurotransmitters as enhancement to the low-phenylalanine diet.

Early treatment with a well-controlled, carefully monitored low-phenylalanine diet has had spectacular results, almost totally eliminating mental retardation in this disease. However, even with early treatment, some children have behavior problems that interfere with learning in school.

Maternal PKU

Through studies of a handful of apparently normal women who inevitably had babies, one after another, with microcephaly, it was found that these women were undiagnosed cases of PKU. They had typically elevated levels of phenylalanine but, for reasons that are not totally clear, were only mildly intellectually handicapped. However, their phenylalanine and its metabolites crossed the placenta during pregnancy and damaged the developing fetal brain even though genetically most of the children were only heterozygous for the mutant allele and under ordinary circumstances would have been developmentally normal.

Currently, all women with PKU are counseled either to stay on the low-phenylalanine diet at least until they have had their children or to go back on the diet before they consider becoming pregnant. The diet is not a very pleasant one since very little natural protein is allowed, and thus, it is extremely difficult for women to go back on the diet for the child-bearing years, hence the advice that they just stay on it.

CONGENITAL HYPOTHYROIDISM

Congenital hypothyroidism is the most frequent metabolic disorder currently detected by newborn screening. The overall incidence is about one in 4,000 births. More than 90% of cases are sporadic, due to thyroid agenesis or ectopia. The cause of those congenital anomalies is unknown. The remaining cases of congenital hypothryoidism are inborn errors of metabolism and include the following:

- Defects in thyroid hormone biosynthesis
- Thyroid hormone resistance
- Anomalies of thyroid stimulating hormone (TSH)
- Abnormality of the TSH receptors
- Deficient thyroid peroxidase activity

The clinical manifestations of untreated hypothyroidism do not usually appear until the infant is weeks to months old, when growth deficiency, delayed neurocognitive development and, in some cases, mental retardation become evident. Physical characteristics include coarsening of facial features, coarse hair, umbilical hernia, and thick doughy-feeling subcutaneous tissues—the clinical picture of **cretinism** (a term that appropriately has fallen into disuse).

The newborn screening test is done on the filter-paper blood spots collected for other metabolic studies and there are two biochemical approaches in general use: primary screen for thyroxine (T4) and primary screen for elevated TSH. Both work equally well.

The treatment is straightforward and consists of oral thyroxine. As long as T4 supplementation is started during the first few weeks of life, it is usually very effective. As one would expect, there is heterogeneity even among the sporadic cases and some of the severely affected infants show a variety of developmental problems in spite of early treatment.

SICKLE CELL ANEMIA

Sickle cell anemia is a common autosomal recessive disease among people of African heritage with an incidence of about one in 400 births. The test for hemoglobin S is also done on the blood spots and is part of newborn screening in the United States but few other places. Many other hemoglobinopathies will be detected as well, but they are all rare. Children with sickle cell anemia suffer from vasculo-occlusive crises and susceptibility to bacterial infections, especially *Streptococcus pneumoniae* and *Haemophilus influenzae*. The red blood cells of the affected individual have increased fragility, leading to hemolytic anemia that can require frequent blood transfusions. Mortality rates are high, especially in the first 6 to 12 months of life, as a result of bacterial infection or acute splenic sequestration.

The justification for screening includes providing an opportunity for prophylactic antibiotic therapy to prevent fatal bacterial infection, along with immunization against pneumococci and *H. influenzae*. The newborn screening programs also avoid delay in diagnosis, thus facilitating prevention of other serious clinical manifestations, for example, those due to acute sporadic sequestration of red cells in the spleen and aplastic crises that occur when red cell production slows, usually during acute infections, especially viral. An additional benefit is the identification of both parents as carriers; some will want to have genetic counseling and might consider the option of prenatal detection for future pregnancies.

There are some problems relevant to sickle cell screening. One of the controversial issues is whether sickle cell screening should be limited to black children. Obviously, that raises questions of discrimination but inclusion of white babies in the screening programs is economically unsound. The question of whether it makes sense to do this type of screening in states with relatively low black populations also has been raised.

GALACTOSEMIA

Galactosemia, another autosomal recessive condition with many variants, is included in blood spot screening in most of the United States. It is relatively rare (birth incidence reported from one in 35,000 to one in 70,000 in various parts of the world), but nevertheless, if untreated, it is a significant cause of mental retardation and neonatal death. In classic galactosemia, affected individuals have impairment of galactose metabolism due to deficient activity of the enzyme galactose-1-phosphate uridyl transferase. Recognizable manifestations usually appear within a few weeks of birth and include failure to thrive, diarrhea, vomiting, and jaundice. Cataracts develop, as does cirrhosis of the liver. Treatment is straightforward: elimination of lactose-containing milk and milk products from the diet. But even with early detection and treatment, affected children often have speech difficulties, problems with both fine and gross motor control, and various degrees of intellectual impairment. Another problem is a unique susceptibility to neonatal *Escherichia coli* septicemia, which has a high mortality rate. Screening for infants with galactosemia thus carries an urgency that is not quite as important as for the other three conditions described above: it requires a *rapid* laboratory turnaround time to be efficacious! The literature is replete with cases of infants who were near death or dead, or severely jaundiced and brain-damaged, with a diagnosis established on the basis of the clinical presentation before the screening laboratory reported a positive screen test!

FUTURE OF NEWBORN SCREENING

To date, screening of newborns for just three diseases, PKU, hypothyroidism, and sickle cell disease, has had a significant impact on the prevention of disease.

Why have we been so limited? Well, a rational approach has been maintained; that is, criteria have been defined and must be fulfilled before a condition is included in a newborn screening program. See if you can come up with at least half a dozen criteria that you think would be essential before reading on. Here they are:

- Condition should be relatively common
- Its manifestations should be clearly defined
- It must be treatable or preventable with an improved health outcome
- Screening process must be widely available, rapid, inexpensive, and accurate (few false positives or false negatives)
- Confirmatory *diagnostic* tests must be available as well as follow-up services for the patient and family
- Screen must achieve acceptance by medical practitioners
- Public must be made aware of the testing through education and informed consent
- Participation should *not* be made mandatory by law

Techniques have been available for several decades that could be applied to newborn screening for many more of the inborn errors of metabolism. Pilot studies have been carried out and in almost all jurisdictions, and expanded newborn screening has been abandoned. The reasons for this include the rarity of the other inborn errors, the absence of effective treatment, and the high cost of most of the additional testing procedures (most are done on cord blood rather than the blood spots and efficient collection is more difficult and more costly).

But a new era is approaching as a result of rapidly developing technology and the completion of the Human Genome Project. Screening will ineluctably expand to cover an increasing number of treatable genetic diseases.

Additional Problems To Keep in Mind

Missed Cases

Home births complicate the problem of collecting the blood spots, and in many areas, availability of public health nurses to do home visits that could include the collection of blood spots has not been developed. Obtaining blood specimens in the doctor's office is, of course, another option but follow-up visits for well babies are often problematic. Furthermore, delays in obtaining the blood spots beyond the first 2 to 3 weeks of life will delay diagnosis and, in many cases, compromise the effectiveness of preventive treatment. Cases missed because of false negatives are now rare and most are the result of laboratory error.

False Positives

Although screening, by definition, will include false positives under any circumstances, this has been the bane of newborn screening. The anxiety produced by having to inform parents of a positive test for a disease that could cause mental retardation is devastating and the time between the false positive and confirmation of a true positive is one of very high anxiety. Even when the test is proven to be a false positive, for many parents lingering anxiety will persist for unknown periods of time and this can be very upsetting. Some will ask, quite appropriately, why we believe the second test rather than the first. Fortunately, the false positive rates for both congenital hypothyroidism and PKU are below 0.05%.

Clinical Scenario: Denouement

The issues arising from the clinical scenario have been addressed. The family physician's initial discussion with Bob and Sal should be optimistic. The family will be referred to a metabolic clinic for the testing procedures that will confirm the diagnosis and identify the specific mutant allele(s) that caused the disease. The treatment will be explained in detail and the special formula prescribed. Follow-up appointments are essential for the careful monitoring of phenylalanine levels and rate of growth, and to provide an ongoing source of information for the family. Assuming that the specific mutation(s) are identified, prenatal diagnosis for future pregnancies is a possibility *but, given the good prognosis for the patient diagnosed early, very few couples with an affected child would consider this.*

LEARNING POINTS

Genetic screening, in general, can be defined as a search in a population for persons with certain genotypes that can cause or predispose to diseases or lead to disease among their descendants.

Newborn genetic screening can be defined as a search for asymptomatic newborn infants who have inherited a disease that through early diagnosis and institution of medical management will have its manifestations either prevented or greatly minimized. Conditions generally screened for among newborns include the following:

- PKU
- Congenital hypothyroidism
- Hemoglobinopathies
- Galactosemia

PKU, although an autosomal recessive disease, shows such heterogeneity that it verges on fulfilling the criteria for a complex disorder. It also exemplifies a general phenomenon for metabolic diseases: a block in a pathway causes three possibly toxic events:

- Excess substrate proximal to the block
- Excess of breakdown metabolites from that substrate
- Deficiency of metabolites distal to the block

Problems to keep in mind relevant to newborn screening are:

- Missed cases, some of which will be a result of the increasing numbers of home births
- False positive tests will occur
- Genetic heterogeneity

*All screening tests must be followed by appropriate **diagnostic** procedures; a positive screening test does not make a diagnosis, it simply indicates a higher risk!*

References

1. Penrose L, Quastel JH. Metabolic studies in phenylketonuria. Biochem J 1937; 31:266.
2. Levy HL, Albers S. Genetic screening of newborns. Annu Rev Genomics Hum Genet 2000;01:139–77.

Further Reading

Guthrie R. Blood screening for phenylketonuria. JAMA 1961;178:863
MacCready RA. Phenylketonuria screening programs. N Engl J Med 1963;269:52.

cells throughout the body, accumulation is limited mainly to the reticuloen-dothelial system. Most affected individuals have some degree of hepatosplenomegaly and occasionally the splenomegaly is so massive that there is a risk of rupture after relatively minor abdominal trauma; hyper-splenism with resultant pancytopenia also can occur. In some cases, bone infiltration by Gaucher's cells (cerebroside-laden reticuloendothelial cells) leads to bone pain. Intellect is unaffected and there are no neurological man-ifestations in type 1 disease. Gaucher's disease is by far the most common of the so-called Jewish diseases with a carrier frequency of approximately one in 16 and thus, an incidence of affected individuals of just over one in 1,000! Molecular methods can provide accurate carrier detection: screening for five mutant alleles allows determination of more than 95% of heterozygotes among Ashkenazi Jews. However, neither the molecular nor the biochemical detection of residual enzyme activity correlates with the severity of the phe-notype and major differences in clinical manifestations have been seen even between monozygous twins. In addition, enzyme replacement therapy is available and has proven effective for many patients, providing relief of bone pain, reduction in liver and spleen size, and restoration of abnormal blood counts. Treatment is costly: $100,000 to $400,000 US per year per patient! Thus, since so many affected individuals are so mildly symptomatic that they are unaware that they have the condition, and those most severely affected can be treated successfully, whether or not to embark on carrier screening has remained highly controversial.

A package of screening tests that includes all four of the above condi-tions plus CF (see below) is available from some laboratories. Laboratory fees range as high as $500 per couple in the United States.

Specific Population Screening for Non-Jewish Couples

Sickle cell disease. The stereotype for sickle cell disease is a black individ-ual with severe chronic hemolytic anemia who has several acute crises each year and a lifespan of some 20 years. However, tremendous variation in the manifestations, even without modern advances in treatment, makes prena-tal diagnosis an issue that requires an up-to-date knowledge of the disease by the physician and careful attention to the education of the at-risk cou-ple. Regarding prenatal diagnosis, carrier screening is available in virtually all clinical laboratories and once a couple is identified as high risk, molec-ular analysis is indicated if prenatal detection is desired. Fetal blood sam-pling is no longer necessary.

β-Thalassemia. β-Thalassemia is, for most affected individuals, a severe, chronic hemolytic anemia. It has increased incidence among people whose origins are in the Mediterranean areas—southern Italy, Greece, Cyprus, and Africa—as well as the Middle East and India. In some communities the carrier frequency reaches as high as one in 10, giving an incidence of approximately one in 400 live births. The treatment is regular blood transfusions and the main complication of that is iron storage disease, which must be treated by injected chelating agents. Although death in childhood still occurs as a result of aplastic bone marrow crises and other complications, lifespan in general has been extended to the early adult years by these therapies, but they have a significant negative effect on lifestyle and the disease is still considered to be lethal. Prenatal diagnosis has been accepted by many of the at-risk populations and as a result, the incidence of the disease has dropped significantly in, for example, Greece and Sardinia.

The current recommendation is that every woman, regardless of ethnic origin, have a prepregnancy mean red cell volume test; if below the normal range, further diagnostic testing would be indicated to establish either β-thalassemia carrier status or simple iron deficiency. Laboratory test results for a typical β-thalassemia carrier are shown in Table 6–1.

Table 6–1
Findings in a Typical β-Thalassemia Carrier

	Mean Cell Volume (fL)	% Hemoglobin A_2	Electrophoresis
Carrier	67	7.0	$A–F–A_2$
Normal range	80–110	1.2–3.5	$A–A_2$

α-Thalassemia. α-Thalassemias are a group of anemias seen primarily among people of Southeast Asian origin (Southern China, the Philippines, Thailand, Laos, Malaysia, Cambodia, Myanmar, and India) and of African descent. However, with increasing immigration of Asian peoples to North America, Europe, and Australia, all physicians must keep this disease in mind and be sure to test potential parents whose origins are in those regions. Genetically, the α-thalassemias are very different from the β-thalassemias because the α-chains of the hemoglobin molecule are the product of four genes (two pairs of alleles) rather than one pair of alleles, as for the β-chains (Figure 6–3, A). Mutations involving one of the alleles causes no clinical effect (Figure 6–3, B). If two of the alleles are mutated, either both on the same chromosome or one on each, there is some reduction of α-chain production and affected individuals have mild anemia with small, underhemoglobinized red cells (Figure 6–3, C). With three of the four alleles mutated (Figure 6–3, D), there is greatly reduced α-chain production and the excess β-chains accumulate to form tetramers (hemoglobin H). Patients have mild to moderate hemolytic anemia and can appear quite similar to individuals with β-thalassemia. In the most severe form,

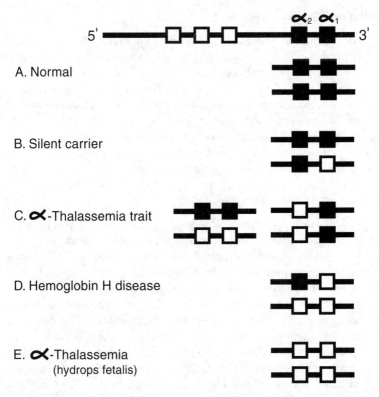

Figure 6–3 *A,* Upper portion represents the α cluster on chromosome 16. The empty boxes are the "α-like" loci and are not transcribed. The transcribing loci are marked α_2 and α_1. The lower portion represents a homozygous normal individual—all four alleles are normal. *B,* One of the four alleles is mutated. There are no clinical consequences; it does not matter whether one of the α_2 or α_1 alleles is mutant. *C,* α-Thalassemia heterozygote. Two of the alleles are mutated. *D,* Hemoglobin H disease. Three of the four alleles are mutated; the excess β-chains form tetramers known as hemoglobin H. *E,* Hemoglobin Bart's. All four α-alleles are mutated. (-■- represents the normal α-chain allele and -□-, a mutated allele.)

hemoglobin Bart's hydrops fetalis, all four α alleles are mutated (Figure 6–3, E) and the condition is lethal: affected fetuses might be stillborn or die shortly after delivery. In China, for example, α-thalassemia is the most common cause of hydrops fetalis. Identification of couples at risk is straightforward and prenatal detection is available in many molecular genetics laboratories. Again, it is important to obtain ethnic histories: increasing numbers of our patients are of mixed racial background and depending on names and physical appearance is unacceptable.

Maternal Serum Screening

Maternal serum screening (MSS), or multiple-marker MSS, is a blood test available to all pregnant women and it is the responsibility of every physician, regardless of his or her personal ethical beliefs, to inform all couples of the availability of this screening test. Brochures, prepared in several languages, are available for both physicians and patients in virtually all areas of North America and many other communities around the world. *Written informed consent is essential.* Every woman must understand that the decision as to whether or not to have such testing is entirely voluntary. The test screens for the disorders described below.

Neural Tube Defects (Spina Bifida)

Neural tube defects (NTDs) are congenital malformations due to failure of the neural groove to close at around the 28th day of fetal development. The incidence in the white population is about one to two per 1,000 live births but it is less common among blacks and Asians. About half the cases of NTDs are **anencephaly** (Figure 6–4) and the rest are **meningoceles**, **meningomyeloceles** (Figure 6–5), and **encephaloceles**. The precise cause of the defects is unknown but there is no question that both genetic and environmental factors play roles; this is a classic multifactorial or complex disorder.

Anencephaly, literally absence of the brain, is uniformly lethal. Much of the cranium is absent and the cerebral hemispheres are severely underdeveloped; the infant is either stillborn or dies within hours. The other NTDs have highly variable manifestations; a meningocele, for example, consists of a sac of cerebrospinal fluid containing no neural elements and usually results in little if any neurological dysfunction. Meningomyeloceles contain neural tissue and impairment of function varies from relatively mild bladder and bowel difficulties to total loss of control, and varying degrees of paralysis, usually from the waist down. Hydrocephalus is a frequent addi-

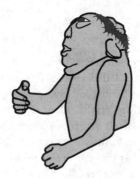

Figure 6–4 Anencephaly showing protruding brain.

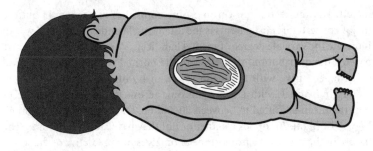

Figure 6–5 Meningomyelocele with bilateral clubfeet.

tional complication that often has a postnatal onset; head circumference must be carefully monitored by ultrasound examinations and regularly scheduled head measurements. With prompt attention to treatment and careful monitoring for complications, physical handicaps can be mitigated or prevented and most affected children, with or without hydrocephalus, are intellectually unimpaired.

It should be emphasized that **spina bifida occulta (SBO)** is a separate minor malformation that is extremely common, with a frequency that is possibly as high as 40% of the population! Most of the time it is noted on X-rays taken for other purposes, such as the investigation of back pain. SBO has nothing to do with NTDs (and doesn't cause back pain either). It is simply a defect in the formation of the vertebral arch; it is a mesenchymal anomaly rather than a defect of the neuroectoderm. The defects in the vertebral arches seen in true NTDs are secondary to the defect in the closure of the neural tube. In SBO, usually one or two arches are affected and a history of SBO in relatives can be ignored. However, when three or more vertebral arches are involved or if there is any history of even mild urinary tract dysfunction, it would be wise to consider that anomaly as a possible NTD—close relatives could be at risk of having children with NTDs; err on the safe side!

Down Syndrome

By far the most common chromosome anomaly, Down syndrome has an overall incidence of one in 600 live births. There is a marked maternal age effect; a rough and easy-to-remember guide to incidence to present to couples is as follows: at age 20, the incidence is about one in **2000**; at age 35, it is one in **350**; and by the 40s, it is one in **40**

The cause of Down syndrome is the presence of extra genetic material from chromosome 21, usually in the form of a whole extra chromosome: trisomy 21. The manifestations are variable in both occurrence and severity (a more detailed description with hints as to how to remember them is included in the section on chromosome anomalies in chapter 1) but the major concern for most parents is the intellectual handicap. A useful way to illustrate the variable degree of mental handicap is to explain to prospective parents the distribution of intellect in the normal population as a typical bell-shaped curve with the mean set at an IQ of 100. IQ is distributed among individuals with Down syndrome in exactly the same way except that the mean is shifted to between 50 and 60. Obviously, some children's IQ will be in the 70s or 80s whether or not they have Down syndrome. The nature of the causative chromosome anomaly is not predictive of the severity of the manifestations.

Trisomy 18 (Edwards' Syndrome)

A relatively rare chromosome anomaly, trisomy 18 has an incidence of approximately one in 3,000 live births and a remarkable sex ratio of three females to one male. The cause of the latter is unknown. The consequences of this anomaly are serious, with developmental delay, both physical and mental. Most infants with trisomy 18 die within weeks to months but survival into the teenage years and even adult life does occur rarely. The characteristic physical signs mostly relate to small features, such as low birth weight, tiny facial structures, and a prominent occiput as seen in premature infants. Heart defects are common and there is often a characteristic overlapping of the index finger onto the 2nd and 3rd fingers. Additional details are presented in the chromosome anomalies section of chapter 1.

Carrier Testing for Other Autosomal Recessive Diseases

Cystic Fibrosis

Although major advances have been made in the treatment of CF, with the majority of individuals who make it out of the neonatal period surviving into their 20s or 30s, it continues to be a very serious and, almost always, an ultimately fatal disease. The basic defect is in the structure of a membrane transport glycoprotein, cystic fibrosis transmembrane conductance regulator (CFTR), responsible for maintenance of the proper concentrations of electrolytes in, among other secretory products, extracellular mucus. The mucoproteins of the CF patient are thickened and as a result, passage of various secretions is impeded (Figure 6–6). A major target is the tracheobronchial system, where plugged respiratory bronchi and bronchioles cause mucus and debris to accumulate distal to the obstructions. The fluids are excellent culture media for bacteria and fungi and hence the repeated episodes of pneumonia and eventually, bronchiectasis. Plugged pancreatic ducts cause rupture of exocrine ductules and acini with spilling of digestive

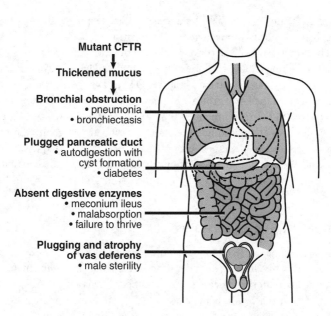

Figure 6–6 Pathogenesis of manifestations of cystic fibrosis. CFTR = cystic fibrosis trans-membrane conductance regulator.

pancreatic enzymes into the tissues of the pancreas. Autodigestion occurs with inflammation, necrosis, and subsequent scarring with cyst formation due to glandular excretions accumulating distal to obstructed ducts; hence the original name of the disease, cystic fibrosis of the pancreas. Failure of digestive enzymes to reach the digestive tracts in the developing fetus can lead to undigested meconium obstructing the bowel and the affected newborn could have the CF manifestation known as **meconium ileus**. There is a high mortality rate associated with that manifestation. In older children with CF, diabetes mellitus often occurs as a result of gradual destruction of the islets of Langerhans as inflammation and scarring spread to the more distal areas of the pancreas. Treatment of CF includes supplements of pancreatic digestive enzymes, antibiotics, and vitamins, along with vigorous respiratory physiotherapy. Literally hundreds of different mutant alleles have been shown to cause CF and some clinical-molecular correlations are emerging. However, about a dozen mutant alleles account for the majority of cases of CF in the North American white population, where the carrier frequency is about one in 20. There is no increased incidence among Jews. In certain other ethnic groups specific alleles account for the majority of cases, as in areas of Sardinia. CF is relatively rare among blacks and Asians. Screening for carrier detection is a problem in most populations. Using the most common alleles for the white population, about 85% of carriers can be identified. Many epidemiologists and geneticists feel that this is not good enough and have discouraged general population screening for carriers.

The American College of Medical Genetics has stated as a policy that carrier screening should be done only for couples where one or both partners has CF or has an affected relative. On the other hand, a consensus statement developed by a group brought together by the US National Institutes of Health has recommended that genetic testing for CF be offered to *all* couples who are planning a pregnancy or who are pregnant, as long as adequate education, genetic counseling, and other support systems are in place and there is adequate experience with sensitivity and specificity of the testing for the mutations for CF in the ethnic and racial groups being served.

Relatively Rare Genetic Diseases

Most of the time the need for screening for rare genetic diseases will arise from a family history that includes a close relative with an inborn error of metabolism or another disease in which either there is a biochemical factor or a mutation that is known and for which there is an available test. The message is: Whenever you find a genetic condition by family history, you must check whether there is biochemical or molecular testing that can detect carriers of recessive disorders or presymptomatic persons with dominant disorders. Consult the Web sites at the end of this chapter or a genetics center.

PROCEDURES FOR THE PRACTICING PHYSICIAN

Tay-Sachs Disease

Blood samples should be obtained from both parents to test for Tay-Sachs disease, preferably before pregnancy occurs. It is essential to indicate on the requisition whether the woman is pregnant and how far along. The serum test will be performed on the father; for the mother the test will be done on leukocytes from a heparinized tube of blood. Results usually are available within a few days. If the couple wishes to have testing for the other "Jewish diseases" plus CF, the physician should consider referral to a genetics center or to one of the special laboratories that offer the screening package (see Web sites at the end of the chapter).

Only when *both* parents are carriers is further action indicated. Special molecular testing is available to confirm that the parents are "true" carriers and to identify the specific mutation(s). The various options must now be discussed or rediscussed with the couple. Prenatal diagnosis by chorionic villus sampling (CVS) or amniocentesis is available and it is imperative to be certain that the couple understands the risk that the fetus will be affected, the risk of the prenatal tests themselves, and the possibility that they will have to face the decision of terminating the pregnancy because there is no way to prevent the disease (see "Ethical Issues" below).

NTDs and Other Congenital Anomalies

If there is any question at all about menstrual dates, a dating ultrasound examination should be done because the timing of subsequent testing is critical. In addition, the presence of more than one fetus will be determined and that would eliminate the possibility of having MSS for chromosome anomalies.

Maternal Serum Screening

The purpose of MSS is to determine whether the fetus is at increased risk of having Down syndrome, trisomy 18, an open NTD, or other anomalies. The serum sample will be assayed for α-fetoprotein (AFP) and other metabolites, most frequently human chorionic gonadotropin (hCG), and unconjugated estriol (uE$_3$), all of which are known to be elevated or decreased in the above conditions. Inhibin-A has been added in some programs with a significantly increased detection rate for Down syndrome (at about US$13 per test, inhibin assay is expensive, but detects about one quarter of the cases of Down syndrome missed with the triple screen without increasing the number of false positives). Computer programs in each laboratory analyze the results in concert with maternal age to determine risk figures for each of the above. Approximate detection rates are 70% for Down syndrome (76% with inhibin-A), 75% for trisomy 18, and 80% for open NTDs.

Again, it must be emphasized that this is a *screening* test: by definition, some affected fetuses will be missed and some normal fetuses will be classified as possibly affected. Pregnant women with insulin-dependent diabetes mellitus should be considered as a separate category. AFP levels are lower, on average, for women with diabetes, and this should be taken into consideration when interpreting results. The flow chart in Figure 6–7 is a summary of the MSS protocol.

The optimal time to obtain the sample for MSS is 15 to 16 weeks' gestation because the test's sensitivity is best at that time.

About eight of every 100 women tested will have a screen positive result; four for NTDs and four for Down syndrome. *This does not mean that the fetus is affected by either.* In fact, most of the fetuses that screen positive are not affected with anything; the positive test result simply indicates an increased risk and further investigations are indicated.

Maternal Serum Screening (MSS) Protocol

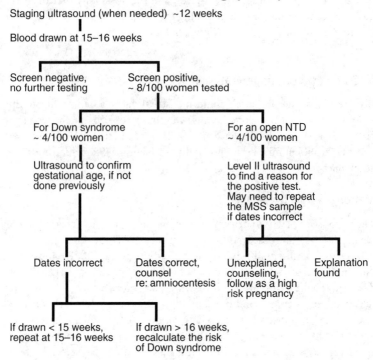

Staging ultrasound (when needed) ~12 weeks

Blood drawn at 15–16 weeks

Screen negative, no further testing

Screen positive, ~ 8/100 women tested

For Down syndrome ~ 4/100 women

For an open NTD ~ 4/100 women

Ultrasound to confirm gestational age, if not done previously

Level II ultrasound to find a reason for the positive test. May need to repeat the MSS sample if dates incorrect

Dates incorrect

Dates correct, counsel re: amniocentesis

Unexplained, counseling, follow as a high risk pregnancy

Explanation found

If drawn < 15 weeks, repeat at 15–16 weeks

If drawn > 16 weeks, recalculate the risk of Down syndrome

Figure 6–7 Maternal serum screening flow chart.

Screen positive results for Down syndrome mean that the chance of the baby being born with that condition is equal to or greater than about one in 350. That risk figure is arbitrary and the cut-off point is set by the laboratory; it is, in fact, about the risk of Down syndrome at maternal age 35 years. A specific risk figure based on a combination of the multiple marker assay results and the maternal age will be reported. Each woman will then have to decide whether to proceed to amniocentesis, the *diagnostic* test for Down syndrome and other chromosome anomalies.

Screen positive results for an open NTD mean that the AFP result is equal to or greater than 2.2 multiples of the median (MOM) and the fetus is at increased risk of having an open NTD. This reporting system was agreed upon internationally so that each laboratory service determines its own set of normal values. The 2.2 MOM has been calculated to maximize detection of open NTDs without an unacceptably high number of false positive results. The use of MOM rather than actual assay levels allows comparison of results among laboratories wherever they might be. About 4% of pregnancies will test positive with the 2.2 MOM cut-off point.

Detailed Fetal Ultrasonography

The next step after a screen positive result for an open NTD is a level II or detailed fetal ultrasound examination ASAP! It should be noted that there are several congenital anomalies in addition to open NTDs that can be associated with a screen positive result and provide unexpected and possibly very upsetting information. Forewarning the patient might be helpful.

The issue of whether *every* pregnant woman should have fetal ultrasonography at 17 to 18 weeks is controversial. Unexpected fetal anomalies, including congenital heart defects, abdominal wall defects, NTDs, and so on, will be detected. However, the incidence of detectable anomalies might not be high enough to justify the enormous cost in dollars plus the anxiety created by positive findings, some of which will include relatively minor or repairable anomalies such as cleft lip, cleft palate, polydactyly, and club feet. On the other hand, although all of the above defects occur as isolated anomalies, they are also frequently found in chromosome anomalies and their detection by ultrasonography becomes an indication for an emergency fetal karyotype. This late in pregnancy, fetal blood aspiration might be required for that purpose.

Keep in mind that by far the most common cause of a screen positive result for open NTDs is a normal pregnancy! As well, there are many multiple malformation syndromes, some genetic and some not, in which an NTD could be one of many manifestations (trisomy 13, Meckel-Gruber syndrome, fetal hydantoin syndrome). In addition, there are other causes for a positive test result. *See if you can come up with a short list of conditions other than NTDs that will result in a screen positive result before reading on.*

Anything that might cause an excessive leak of fetal serum into the amniotic fluid and from there into the maternal circulation can lead to a positive result. Examples include omphalocele or gastroschisis (i.e., ventral abdominal wall defects), cystic hygroma, any bullous skin lesion (e.g., epidermolysis bullosa), more than one fetus, fetal death, and congenital nephrosis (flow of fetal protein-laden urine into the amniotic fluid).

In any case, an *unexplained* positive MSS for NTDs requires that the pregnancy be considered high risk and monitored carefully for its entirety. Many geneticists and obstetricians recommend amniocentesis in all such cases.

Alternate Clinical Scenario: Advanced Maternal Age

Suppose Mrs. Sampson is 38 years old. What do think the difference in approach would be?

Any pregnant woman who will be 35 or older at the estimated date of confinement is considered to be at high risk of carrying a fetus with a chromosome anomaly, especially trisomy 21, and therefore eligible for a diagnostic prenatal test—CVS or amniocentesis.

The only important issue from the genetic point of view is whether or not to do the MSS for identifying pregnancies at increased risk for a fetus with a trisomy. As noted above, the risk for Down syndrome increases with advancing maternal age. NTDs, other anatomical defects, and metabolic diseases do not show a maternal age effect. What about other chromosome anomalies? There is a slight maternal age effect for the sex chromosome anomalies (e.g., 47,XXY; 47,XXX) and also for the other autosomal trisomies, but the increase is nowhere near as marked as for trisomy 21.

Some women from ages 35 to 38 or 39 who are uncertain as to whether to undergo amniocentesis elect to have MSS. If the result drops their risk to that of a woman younger than themselves, they might elect not to proceed with the invasive test. Many geneticists and obstetricians agree that MSS has no place in the management of pregnancy in a woman over 39 simply because the risk of a fetal chromosome anomaly is too high just on the basis of maternal age.

An important point to keep in mind is that the woman who undergoes CVS at 10 to12 weeks' gestation must consider having MSS at 15 to 17 weeks because of the remaining possibility of an NTD or other detectable congenital anomalies. In addition, the indications for fetal ultrasonography would remain unchanged, except that the chromosome analysis would have excluded those conditions.

Is there a *paternal* age effect? Yes, but it is small enough to safely ignore. For example, for a 34-year-old woman to qualify for amniocentesis on the basis of advanced maternal age, the father would have to be near 60 to move her risk up to that of a 35-year-old woman. A much better approach would, of course, be MSS.

First-Trimester Screening for Fetal Anomalies

Studies are underway to determine the feasibility of screening between 10 and 13 weeks' gestation with a combination of biochemical markers and ultrasonography. Early results using the biochemical markers **p**regnancy-**a**ssociated **p**lasma **p**rotein-A (PAPP-A) and free β-hCG together with nuchal translucency measurements by ultrasonography (see chapter 3, Figure 3–29) have shown a remarkable 85% detection rate for Down syndrome with a 5% false positive rate. Emerging is a recommendation for what is being referred to as the **integrated test** combining results from screening for both first- and second-trimester markers; this is providing a detection rate of approximately 94% with a 5% false positive rate.

In addition, first-trimester fetal ultrasonography, because of newer technology providing better resolution and even three-dimensional images, could be useful in the early detection of anomalies other than Down syndrome. Examples include central nervous system anomalies, such as anen-

lence and confusion; genetic counseling services are available and genetic counselors are well equipped to present both sides of the various issues. In addition, these issues are being taught and discussed by most religious groups; referral to the clergy might be very helpful for some couples.

Although patient-oriented brochures on nearly all aspects of prenatal diagnosis are available in many languages, along with videotapes and other explanatory documents, the physician cannot rely on these alone. Illiteracy rates in virtually all populations are surprisingly high and every woman or couple contemplating any type of prenatal diagnosis must be given the opportunity to discuss the issues and to ask questions directly of the physician or a well-informed, well-trained health care professional assistant. There should never be any hesitation to refer to a genetics clinic.

Furthermore, it is the responsibility of every physician who provides care for pregnant women to, at the very least, inform them of the availability of prenatal diagnostic techniques regardless of his or her own moral beliefs and ethical practices. Obviously, no physician is under any obligation to actually provide the necessary procedures; the patient can be referred to other physicians or clinics. On the other hand, prenatal diagnosis has been clearly established as a standard of care nationally and internationally and unfortunately, lawsuits regarding these aspects of health care are becoming increasingly common. Ignorance of new developments is not a valid defense strategy.

Under no circumstances should any prenatal screening or diagnostic procedure be undertaken without written informed consent. Consent forms are available from all genetics clinics and most obstetrical units.

Finally, the physician must be prepared to deal with the issue of false paternity. Molecular genetics laboratories have discovered that close to 1 in 10 "sociologic" fathers is not the biological father, and one large survey indicated a false paternity rate of one in seven! There are many ways for the physician to deal with the problem, including nondisclosure when that knowledge would be of no clinical consequence. However, consultation with a geneticist is highly recommended; this issue is arising with increasing frequency as the number of DNA analyses for screening purposes escalates. The expert advice of the genetics center should be helpful to the practicing doctor.

LEARNING POINTS

Genetic Testing Available for Pregnant Women

- Before becoming pregnant, there should be a thorough discussion of prenatal testing available to all women, as well as special procedures that are indicated as a result of issues that emerge from the family history.

Carrier testing of both parents for CF and any other recessive conditions is best done before the woman is pregnant.

- If the woman is not on folic acid supplementation, it should be started immediately (0.4 mg/day; 4.0 mg/day if there's been a previous child with an NTD).
- 8 to 12 weeks. Staging ultrasound examination for confirmation of menstrual dating of pregnancy (optional).
- 11 to 12 weeks. CVS in cases of advanced maternal age or high risk for chromosomal or metabolic disease, as determined from the family history.
- 10 to 13 weeks. Watch for developments in first trimester detection of Down syndrome and other congenital anomalies using biochemical markers and fetal ultrasonography.
- 14 to 17 weeks. Amniocentesis when indicated, usually in cases of advanced maternal age, a positive multiple-marker MSS test, or an anomaly detected by ultrasonography.
- 17 to 18 weeks. Detailed or level 2 fetal ultrasonography for the detection of fetal anomalies.

Carrier Testing for Specific Ethnic or Racial Groups

- Ashkenazi Jews. Tay-Sachs disease, Canavan's disease, Niemann-Pick disease, and Gaucher's disease; CF testing is optional.
- Individuals of Mediterranean, African, Indian, or Middle Eastern origins. β-Thalassemia.
- People from India, China, and Southeast Asian countries. α-Thalassemia.
- Couples of European descent. Possibly CF.

Advanced Maternal Age (Age 35 or More on Due Date)

- 35 to 38 weeks. Some might consider multiple-marker MSS.
- 39 + weeks. CVS or amniocentesis (this approach can be modified when first-trimester prenatal diagnosis becomes widely available).

Further Reading

Adinolfi M, Sherlock J. First trimester prenatal diagnosis using transcervical cells: an evaluation. Hum Reprod Update 1997;3:383–92.

Carroll JC. Maternal serum screening. Can Fam Physician 1994;40:1756–64.

Dumars KW, Boehm C, Eckman JR, et al. Practical guide to the diagnosis of thalassemia. Council of Regional Networks for Genetic Services (CORN). Am J Med Genet 1996;62:29–37.

Kronn D, Jansen V, Ostrer H. Carrier screening for cystic fibrosis, Gaucher disease, and Tay-Sachs disease in the Ashkenazi Jewish population: the first 1000 cases at New York University Medical Center, New York, NY. Arch Intern Med 1998;158:777–81.

Matalon R. Canavan disease: diagnosis and molecular analysis. Genet Test 1997;1:21–5.

National Institutes of Health Consensus Development Conference Statement on genetic testing for cystic fibrosis. Arch Intern Med 1999;159:1529–39.

Pertl B, Kopp S, Kroisel PM, et al. Rapid detection of chromosome aneuploidies by quantitative fluorescence PCR: first application on 247 chorionic villus samples. J Med Genet 1999;36:300–3.

Policy statement from the American College of Medical Genetics. Folic acid and pregnancy. www.faseb.org/genetics/acmg/pol-menu.htm

Schuchman EH, Miranda SR. Niemann-Pick disease: mutation update, genotype/phenotype correlations, and prospects for genetic testing. Genet Test 1997;1:13–29.

Web Sites

Excellent descriptions of genetic disorders; overviews of basic genetic principles; guide to support groups, genetic counseling, and genetic testing.

GeneClinics   <www.geneclinics.org>

Another excellent source of descriptions of genetic disorders to complement Gene Sage. Neither site is complete; both are expanding rapidly as new conditions are added regularly.

GeneTests   <www.genetests.org>

Data on available genetic testing, including cytogenetic, biochemical, and molecular tests; the laboratories that are able to carry out the required testing both on a clinical or research basis; the genetic counseling center near you; and much more.

Bone Dysplasias and Short Stature

Prologue

What, I hear you ask, is a chapter on an apparently esoteric, or at least a rather specialized, subject doing in a short book for medical students? Well, it's actually not so esoteric and although the details of etiology, diagnosis, and management do indeed dwell in the realm of the specialist, the issues raised are important for every physician. And, by the way, the problem is not so uncommon—if we add up the incidences of the various types of genetically determined dwarfism, they come to between one in 5,000 and one in 6,000 (that's about twice the incidence of phenylketonuria)—and then add in the children who have perfectly normal bones but who are significantly shorter than average!

Clinical Scenario

A 30-year-old woman is in the 17th week of her first pregnancy. There is nothing in her medical or family history to suggest that the pregnancy might be high risk and her maternal serum screening (MSS) test results were reported as screen negative. She was referred for routine level II fetal ultrasonography and the radiologist has just called to tell you that the fetus appears to have a form of short-limbed dwarfism: all four limbs are short in relation to both gestational age and the overall length of the fetus, and the head size is relatively large, although not outside the normal range. Fortunately, both parents are present and, as would be expected, extremely upset and in tears. You tell the radiologist that you will leave for the hospital immediately.

What ought to be going through your mind as you drive the few blocks to the Radiology Department? Before reading on, see if you can jot down what further investigations are indicated, what is the most likely diagnosis, and how are you going to comfort the couple?

Investigations

You would first want to see the ultrasound films yourself and talk to the radiologist. The severity of the limb shortening, which segment is more affected, proximal or distal, and thoracic circumference are very important. In addition, it is essential to assess the presence or absence of intrauterine growth retardation—that could help distinguish a skeletal dysplasia from a syndrome.

Did you think of the need to look carefully for any additional skeletal anomalies, as well as anomalies in other anatomical structures? You might not have known that careful examination of the fingers and toes for the presence of polydactyly can provide a major diagnostic clue (if you got that one, you really did well!). Such findings as a heart defect, kidney anomaly, neural tube defect, and so on would be suggestive of short limbs in association with a chromosome anomaly or a multiple malformation syndrome rather than a primary bone dysplasia. Obtaining a consultation with a pediatric radiologist with special expertise in the bone dysplasias is always indicated.

Diagnostic Hypotheses

Let's assume that no additional structural defects can be detected on the ultrasonogram and the radiologists cannot discern any specific rib, pelvic, or other structural defects. The limb shortening is significant and appears to be primarily proximal, and the overall growth retardation is minimal. Did you come up with achondroplasia as a likely diagnosis? Well, although achondroplasia is by far the most common bone dysplasia syndrome detectable *at birth*, it is probably *not* the correct diagnosis here because the limb shortening and other manifestations of that condition are usually not of sufficient degree to be detectable much before the third trimester. More likely, is one of the lethal bone dysplasias, the most common of which will be described below, along with specific diagnostic tests, some of which are available prenatally.

Counseling

Now you need to think about those frantic parents! The points to discuss in this first session are as follows:

Although a specific diagnosis has not yet been made, the radiological signs are suggestive of one of the types of bone abnormalities that are not compatible with survival after delivery, although the pregnancy, if uninterrupted, could go to term or close to it. In other words, the couple will almost certainly not have a child with severe short stature, mental retardation, and other birth defects. Facing a near-certain loss of the pregnancy will be devastating but the almost certain lethality of the condition might be some small comfort. The importance of sympathetically presenting the option of continuing the pregnancy to term in spite of the inevitable outcome is discussed in chapter 1—you might want to reread it (or read it for the first time!) at this point and keep it in mind whenever you counsel a couple who have to consider termination for any lethal genetic disorder.

Consultation will probably provide a specific diagnosis within a short period of time and a complete explanation of what has happened, including accurate prognosis and risk of recurrence in future pregnancies, will be forthcoming. In addition to expert evaluation of the skeletal system, the specific mutations responsible for many of the bone dysplasias are known and can be determined from molecular testing of fetal cells obtained prenatally. It *is* possible, although unlikely, that you have detected a fetus with achondroplasia and that condition is not lethal. Since it is the most common of the bone dysplasias, we will consider the issues it raises in some detail as a prototype of genetically determined short stature.

Genetic Counseling

While the parents are suffering through the pain and wondering, Why us?, they will inevitably go on to, What next? No one in our family ever had a child who is a dwarf and look at us; we're both *taller* than average—are we likely to have more dwarfed offspring? Well, even before you have any idea as to the specific diagnosis, you can at least begin to reassure them that recurrence risks are very low for *almost* all forms of genetic dwarfism, as we will discuss below.

ACHONDROPLASIA

The incidence of achondroplasia is approximately 1 in 15,000 live births. Clinical features (Figure 7–1) are as follows:

- Disproportionate short stature (mean adult heights are 130 cm for men and 125 cm for women) with rhizomelic shortening of the limbs and marked lumbar kyphosis (sway back)
- Large elongated head with prominent forehead and midfacial hypoplasia
- So-called trident hand where the first two fingers and the 4th and 5th fingers tend to be held close together and with the thumb make a three-sectioned hand, as shown in the right hand of the child in Figure 7–1
- Generalized ligamentous laxity or hyperextensible joints

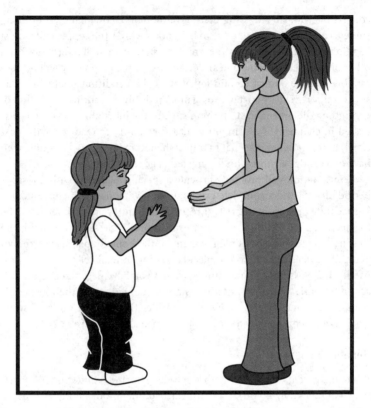

Figure 7–1 A child with achondroplasia. Note the typical head shape, small chest, marked lordosis, and trident hand.

- Genu varum
- Mild to moderate hypotonia in infancy, which, along with the ligamentous laxity, accounts for the delays in achieving motor milestones
- Normal intellect

Complications include the following:

- Sleep apnea in infancy, either obstructive (could be secondary to the midface hypoplasia) or central (brain stem compression)
- Obesity
- Increased risk of sudden infant death syndrome (SIDS) that is probably related to the large head and cervical hypotonia with dislocation of cervical vertebrae and subsequent spinal cord or brain stem compression
- Increased risk of hydrocephalus due to compression of the brain stem as it passes through the relatively small foramen magnum that is characteristic of achondroplasia

The more severe thanatophoric dysplasia (see below) and the less severe hypochondroplasia are also associated with mutations in the receptor 3 gene but in different domains of the molecule. To make matters a bit more complicated, *FGFR3* also plays a role in the signal transduction pathways that apparently mediate longitudinal growth of the endochondral growth plate. There is a complex group of interactions with parathyroid protein receptor function, one of which is to inhibit expression of Indian hedgehog (see "Transcription Factors and Signaling Molecules" in chapter 1), one of the transcription factors. The result is accelerated terminal differentiation to hypertrophic chondrocytes and a shortened growth plate, obviously contributing further to the phenotype.

Now, let us return to the clinical scenario.

The consulting radiologist agrees that this fetus most likely has one of the lethal bone dysplasias. The next step could be amniocentesis to obtain fetal cells for karyotype and DNA assay, although experienced pediatric radiologists will often be able to recommend skipping this step and waiting for either the abortus or the delivered fetus close to or at term.

Achondroplasia will be almost totally ruled out by failure to find either of the typical *FGFR3* mutations, along with the fact that detection of that condition at 17 weeks' gestation is so uncommon. Post-termination or post-natal radiographs or DNA analysis will almost always establish a specific diagnosis. In the unlikely event that the fetus is found to have achondroplasia, the parents might consider continuing the pregnancy after appropriate counseling, wherein the various manifestations of the condition are carefully and honestly presented. Much more likely, the fetus will turn out to have one of the severe and probably lethal bone dysplasias (see below). The specific mutation has been characterized for many of these, and termination of the pregnancy would be an option to consider seriously.

Differential Diagnoses

The differential diagnoses of the short-limbed dysplasias likely to be detected in the second trimester, in order of frequency, are as follows:

Thanatophoric Dysplasia

The word **thanatophoric** does not have a very pleasant origin: *thanatos* is the Greek word for death; *phoria* the term for attraction, leading toward. The incidence of thanatophoric dysplasia is about one in 20,000 births. Clinically, it is like very severe achondroplasia; Figure 7–5 illustrates some of the features. The head is disproportionately large with marked frontal bossing and severe midface hypoplasia. Some patients have a typical cloverleaf skull deformity. There is extreme micromelia of all segments, often with bending; the ribs are short and the chest cavity very small; vertebral bodies are greatly reduced in height with wide intervertebral spaces and

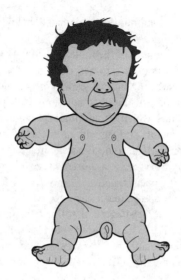

Figure 7–5 Thanatophoric dysplasia.

they might appear horseshoe or H-shaped on ultrasound examination and X-ray. Hydrops fetalis of varying degrees of severity occurs frequently. Death is secondary to pulmonary hypoplasia. Thanatophoria is caused by a group of distinct mutations in *FGFR3*, all of which are different from those found in achondroplasia, and all are present in the heterozygous state. No mutations have been detected in parental DNA, indicating the sporadic nature of this lethal bone dysplasia; proven recurrences in subsequent pregnancies have not been reported.

Achondrogenesis

This is a group of lethal bone dysplasia syndromes characterized by extremely short limbs with a head that is normal sized but appears disproportionately large because of the short trunk and legs, as shown in Figure 7–6. Most patients are hydropic and a striking feature is the marked and generalized deficiency of ossification, most notable in the spine—sometimes the skeletal structures are barely visible on ultrasonograms and X-rays. All patients are either stillborn or suffer early neonatal death. There is clinical and genetic heterogeneity, but the mode of inheritance is autosomal recessive. The most common form is achondrogenesis type 2, which is caused by a new mutation in the gene for type 2 procollagen (*COL2A1*). Specific mutations are being worked out for the other types and molecular diagnosis is not yet available other than for types 2 and 1B. However, the appearance of the fetus on ultrasonograms is nearly always sufficiently characteristic for the prenatal diagnosis to be made.

Diagnosis is based on isolation of the virus from urine or cerebrospinal fluid, and sometimes intracranial distribution of calcium deposition is characteristic.

Herpes simplex. Herpes simplex-1 causes herpes labialis and keratitis and HSV-2 causes herpes labialis, which is transmitted primarily by contact with the lesions. Infection is usually acquired at birth and is often a severe neonatal problem. Intrauterine infection can occur but is extremely rare and is usually due to HSV-2. When it occurs, it is usually lethal because of the severity of the anomalies. All are associated with primary maternal infection during pregnancy. A few neonates have survived with skin lesions and dermatological scars at birth, chorioretinitis, microcephaly or hydranencephaly, and microphthalmia. The rare surviving infants usually have severe CNS sequelae with or without blindness. Nevertheless, because of the rarity of survivors of fetal infection, maternal herpes is not generally considered to be an indication for consideration of abortion.

So much for the TORCH group. Are there any other infectious agents that can cause birth defects? Yes, but only a couple.

Varicella Zoster Virus

Varicella zoster (VZV) infection (chickenpox) is such a highly contagious disease that by age 10, 80% of children have experienced it. Of adults who say that they haven't had chicken pox, more than 85% are seropositive for anti-VZV antibodies. However, roughly one in every 1,500 pregnancies is complicated by maternal chickenpox. The embryopathy can be serious:

- IUGR with limb hypoplasia
- Eye anomalies (cataracts, microphthalmia, chorioretinitis)
- Neurological disorders (microcephaly/cortical atrophy, mental retardation, bowel and bladder sphincter dysfunction)
- Skin scarring

How high is the risk? If the infection occurs in the first 20 weeks of pregnancy, the risk of anomalies is just over 2%.

Pregnancy management. If the pregnant woman is unsure of having had chickenpox as a child, there is a rapid and simple latex agglutination test to measure VZV antibodies. If the test is negative or if for some reason it cannot be obtained, varicella zoster immunoglobulin (VZIG) should be given *within 96 hours of exposure*; one dose is sufficient. Testing with turnaround times of a week or more will *not* be of much help! Studies are ongoing at the time of writing as to the efficacy and safety of VZIG; there have been no reports of fetal embryopathy in any VZIG-treated pregnancy so far.

Maternal Drugs

In general, it is extremely difficult to determine whether drugs have an effect on the embryo or fetus for several reasons. See how many of the possible confounding factors you can think of before going on. OK, here we go.

1. **Timing of ingestion**. The timing of ingestion in relation to gestational age is important; we've already covered this issue.
2. **Numerical risks**. Numerical risks have to be looked at in comparison with the risk of having a child with a birth defect when *no* exposure to teratogens occurred; that is, keep in mind that the incidence of fairly major *congenital* malformations and other genetically determined disorders in the general population is 2% to 3% (that's about one in 30 babies) and by age 7 years, the number rises to 8% to 9% as anomalies that were present at birth but not recognizable are detected (abnormalities of teeth are an obvious example, as are intellectual handicaps).

    When trying to assess the risk of mental handicap, great caution must be used. The socioeconomic status of the family and the IQs of parents and siblings need to be taken into account, as does the average length of follow-up; problems with intellectual function might not become evident until the child is in school and being academically challenged.
3. **Study type**. The type of study reporting a drug as teratogenic is crucial. Retrospective studies are always hazardous because women who have children with anomalies will review the pregnancy looking for anything they might have done to cause the problem, in contrast to those who have normal children. Chart reviews working from infants with specific anomalies to record drugs ingested are fallible for the same reason: too many numerators without very well-documented denominators. Prospective studies are also difficult because of the low incidence of many *specific* congenital anomalies; Ebstein's anomaly of the heart, for example, has an incidence of about one in 20,000 live births. If the drug in question quadrupled the incidence, you'd still have only one affected infant in 5,000 births and it would take quite a study to pick that up!
4. **Brochures**. The brochures prepared by the pharmaceutical company and included with drugs are usually of no help whatsoever, as mentioned previously.

The bottom line: you will need all your critical appraisal skills to assess whatever information you are able to find. *Never* tell a woman that *any* drug is safe during pregnancy before checking it out and even after that, take care with your wording. Let's look at some specific drugs.

Chemotherapeutic Agents

A wide variety of congenital anomalies, most of which are severe, can be expected in anywhere from 7% to 75% of pregnancies when chemotherapeutic drugs are taken in the first half of pregnancy. Other than fetal ultrasonography, there is no prenatal diagnostic test; termination of pregnancy is always an option, sometimes prior to the initiation of chemotherapy if a malignancy requiring such treatment is diagnosed while the woman is pregnant. Supplementary folic acid (4 mg/day) for women requiring antifolates such as methotrexate, might reduce the risk of an adverse fetal outcome for those women who elect to continue a pregnancy. The risk of malformations is not the issue in the second half of pregnancy but prematurity and fetal hemorrhagic disease are. Malformations due to chemotherapeutic drugs could involve virtually all organs and tissues but IUGR and CNS and heart anomalies are the most common.

Anticonvulsants

Attention was first drawn to this group of teratogens by hydantoin (Dilantin) and the **fetal hydantoin syndrome** (FHS) is now a well-established phenomenon. The manifestations include the following:

- Head and facial anomalies such as flat nasal bridge, epicanthal folds; ptosis, strabismus, hypertelorism; low-set or abnormally shaped ears; wide mouth, cleft lip, cleft palate; large fontanelles; microcephaly, mental retardation
- IUGR and postnatal growth retardation
- Cardiac anomalies
- Neuroblastoma

The typical syndrome occurs in 5% to 10% of liveborn infants and some of the manifestations—partial FHS—occur in up to 30% of children of mothers using hydantoin. The risk of intellectual handicap is probably less than 10%.

Carbamazepine. Prospective studies are in progress and so far, the risk of fetal anomalies with carbamazepine (Tegretol) is clearly less than for hydantoin; there have been no reported cases of neuroblastoma or cognitive defects. However, some liveborn infants have had facial characteristics similar to those of patients with FHS and there have been reports of an increased risk of eye anomalies (anophthalmia or microphthalmia, optic disc coloboma) and a probable risk of about 1% for NTDs. Nevertheless, carbamazepine is considered to be the safest of the effective anticonvulsant drugs.

Valproate. The main congenital anomalies associated with valproate are NTDs and the risk is between 1% and 2%.

The bottom line: there is no anticonvulsant or combinations of anticonvulsants for which there is no increased risk of congenital malformations in the fetus when the drug or drugs are taken during the first half of pregnancy.

Pregnancy management for the epileptic woman. Make sure that the patient still requires anticonvulsant therapy. You will be surprised at how often patients remain on anticonvulsants when they haven't had a seizure in years! In consultation with the physician managing the seizure disorder, it might be possible to wean the woman off the drug completely or at least through the first half of the pregnancy. Curiously, lowering the dose of the anticonvulsant rarely makes any difference in relation to teratogenic potential and, in fact, it might be necessary to *increase* the dose during pregnancy because of hemodilution and weight gain in the mother. Monitoring *blood* levels of the drugs is important during pregnancy.

Seizures during pregnancy. Although it might be safer for the fetus to allow an occasional seizure during pregnancy rather than expose it to an anticonvulsant drug, seizures themselves have been implicated as increasing the incidence of congenital anomalies. The reason for that is unknown but hypoxia secondary to the seizure could be a factor.

If possible, switch the mother from multiple- to **single-drug therapy** and try to make the single drug carbamazepine, the anticonvulsant with the lowest risk for serious fetal anomalies, especially cognitive defects. The pregnancy should be monitored by fetal ultrasonography to look for NTDs.

Fetal ultrasound. Serial fetal ultrasound examinations, starting at 17 to 18 weeks, are important for those women on any anticonvulsant who wish to have prenatal detection of such malformations as NTDs, macro- or hydrocephaly, IUGR, and heart defects. Unfortunately, microcephaly is rarely, if ever, severe enough during the first half of pregnancy to be detectable, and hydrocephalus might not become evident until it is too late for intervention.

Diagnostic prenatal testing. Neither **amniocentesis** nor **CVS** would be indicated for women on anticonvulsants except under special circumstances such as advanced maternal age, or an anomaly detected by fetal ultrasonography (chromosome anomalies obviously can occur among epileptic women by chance and finding that as the cause of the detected defect could have a major effect on the prognosis for the affected fetus).

Anxiety. Anxiety is high during any pregnancy and much more so when the mother realizes her epilepsy is putting the fetus at extra risk. Reassurance is essential, emphasizing that, with rare exceptions, anticonvulsants have a deleterious effect on only a minority of exposed fetuses and often a very small minority, especially when considering the most serious defects.

Anticoagulants

Warfarin (coumadin) is the concern here. Fetal warfarin syndrome consists of the following:

- Nasal hypoplasia (the nose can be very tiny and flattened) (see chapter 3, Figure 3–16)
- Chondrodystrophia punctata (punctate skeletal dysplasia) and other skeletal anomalies, including skull defects
- Brachydactyly
- External ear anomalies
- Eye defects; for example, optic atrophy
- Brain anomalies, such as microcephaly, hydrocephaly, the Dandy-Walker anomaly, and spasticity

The risk to the fetus when the mother is on warfarin during the first half of pregnancy is high: 8% of babies are stillborn and about 16% have features of fetal warfarin syndrome. The syndrome is a phenocopy of the relatively rare inherited bone dysplasia, chondrodysplasia punctata (see chapter 7).

Pregnancy management. For a patient on warfarin, pregnancy management begins with trying to switch to heparin *before* the pregnancy occurs. Heparin is not teratogenic, as far as is known, and should be used until midterm. It should be reinstituted near term if anticoagulation is still necessary; the risk of severe and difficult-to-control bleeding is reduced by elective cesarean section for delivery. Obviously, the patient should be followed closely as a high-risk pregnancy.

Sex Hormones

The only *exogenous* sex steroids of concern were those used in oral contraceptives and "were" is used advisedly. Some studies suggested an increased risk of congenital heart defects as a result of these hormones. This observation has *not* stood the test of time, or the risk of a heart defect is so slightly increased that it is barely measurable. No cognitive defects or any other malformations have been documented among the very large study groups of women inadvertently continuing to take oral contraceptive pills for many weeks after becoming pregnant and not realizing it. Reassurance is essential, along with follow-up with fetal ultrasonography to detect a heart defect in the unlikely event of occurrence. Keep in mind that some sort of congenital heart defect occurs spontaneously in close to one per 100 live births.

The bottom line: the use of sex hormones as contraceptives or in creams or other external vehicles does not cause any interference with fetal sex differentiation, nor do they cause birth defects of other kinds, as far as can be detected.

The *endogenous* over- or underproduction of sex hormone precursors, on the other hand, does lead to pseudohermaphroditism and the most common cause of that is fetal adrenal hyperplasia (see chapter 4, "Ambiguous Genitalia").

Tranquilizers and Antidepressants

The widespread use and abuse of tranquilizers and antidepressants make this issue extremely important. The last thing the physician wants to do is make an already anxious patient who is on one of these medications before realizing she is pregnant, even more anxious because of possible risk of the drug causing birth defects. Since close to half of all pregnancies are unplanned, stopping intake of the drug before embarking on a pregnancy is not a very practical solution to the problem. In addition, a sizable proportion of women on these medications benefit greatly from them and stopping taking the medication during a pregnancy or even for half of a pregnancy is not an attractive alternative.

How risky are these drugs? For **lithium**, reports indicated an increased risk of congenital heart defects, especially the rare Ebstein's anomaly (downward displacement of a deformed tricuspid valve with tricuspid regurgitation). If this is true, the magnitude of the increased risk is very small and recent studies have not been able to corroborate the increased risk at all. Furthermore, there is no detectable increased risk of other anomalies or of intellectual developmental deficits. The drug can be continued and the pregnancy monitored by fetal ultrasonography, mainly for reassurance of the parents.

For the **tricyclics, fluoxetine** (Prozac), and **benzodiazepines** (e.g., Valium), none of the substantive studies has established any increased risk of fetal anomalies or interference with intellectual development. Reports of an increased risk of facial clefts (lip or palate) have not been confirmed.

Vitamin A Derivatives

Vitamin A derivatives include isotretinoin (Accutane), tretinoin, and retinoids. *Never has a drug been put on the market with such care regarding the risk of teratogenicity.* Oral isotretinoin was introduced in the early 1980s for the treatment of severe cystic acne. At that time it was known to be teratogenic from studies in laboratory animals and it came on the market as *contraindicated* for women who were or might become pregnant during therapy and in the month following therapy. A Pregnancy Prevention Program was developed by the manufacturer and the US FDA that included printed material for physicians to facilitate patient education. In addition there were instructions to obtain a negative pregnancy test before prescribing the drug and to delay therapy until the second or third day of the next normal menstrual period. The program strongly suggests simultaneous use of two forms of contraception throughout the course of therapy to further reduce the risk of inadvertent fetal exposure. In addition, women were to be asked to sign a consent form acknowledging that they had been instructed through the Pregnancy Prevention Program, that they were aware of the need for contraception during treatment, and that they would undergo pregnancy testing before, during, and after therapy. Nevertheless, the best prevention program ever devised will not work if physicians and patients do not comply and that is exactly what has happened. Cases of isotretinoin embryopathy occurred soon after the drugs were put on the market and they continue to occur with frightening frequency! This group of drugs is among the most potent teratogens known.

Don't let it happen to you. Rigorous attention to prevention is virtually mandated! You will be a sitting duck for a malpractice suit if you do not take the above precautions to reduce the possibility of fetal exposure.

Retinoic acid embryopathy includes anomalies of the central nervous system (hydrocephalus, microcephaly), heart, craniofacial structures, and thymus. The incidence of the embryopathy is close to 40% and of the malformations, 80% involve the CNS. In follow-up studies to 5 years of age, cognitive deficits have been documented in more than half of the children exposed in utero and they often occur in the absence of dysmorphology.

The topical preparations of tretinoin (Retin-A, Renova) are used mainly for the treatment of acne and occasionally for photodamage to the skin. Although no teratogenic effects have been reported in pregnant women, the US Pharmacopoeia Dispensing Information states that topical tretinoin should not be used during pregnancy. Acne is common among women in the childbearing age group and symptomatic treatment with tretinoin is frequent. However, studies have been relatively small and need to be continued and better defined (e.g., better control of concentrations of the active ingredient, better documentation of gestational ages at the times of exposure, inclusion of abortion rates). Again, at this time, inadvertent use of topical retinoids in the first trimester would not be considered an indication for termination of pregnancy; there have been no reports indicating any increased risk of anomalies of any type and certainly no reports of retinoic acid embryopathy.

Antibiotics

The general statement that can be made on data available at the time is that there is no evidence of teratogenicity for antibiotics given at any time during pregnancy. Even the tetracyclines have been overestimated as teratogens and, in fact, don't really qualify; the main effect is yellow-brown discoloration of the teeth caused by antibiotic deposition during calcification. The risk is only *after* 4 to 5 months' gestation, when the deciduous teeth begin to calcify. There could be some deposition in calcifying bone but there have been no reports of any interference in bone formation or growth in humans.

The caveat: new antibiotics appear on the market frequently and new reports on older ones will be published regularly.

Recreational Drugs

Alcohol

Fetal alcohol syndrome (FAS), completely defined in 1973, includes the following main features:

- Growth retardation (low birth weight, decelerating weight gain over time, or both, not due to malnutrition)
- Characteristic facial anomalies: short palpebral fissures and anomalous development of the premaxillary zone (long upper lip, flat midface with a flat philtrum)
- CNS anomalies: microcephaly, partial or complete agenesis of the corpus callosum, impaired fine motor skills, poor hand–eye coordination, neurosensory hearing loss, delayed language development, and behavioral aberrations
- Increased incidence of other congenital anomalies involving heart, skeleton, kidneys, and eyes

The risk of having a child with some or most of the manifestations of FAS for a given individual who drinks during a pregnancy is impossible to predict. As noted in the introduction to this chapter, although the timing and amount of the maternal alcohol intake are important, a host of additional factors plays a role. There is no question that alcohol has a deleterious effect on the fetus, and the damage can occur at any and all times throughout the entire gestational period, as would be expected. The incidence of liveborn infants with **fetal alcohol effects** (some of the signs of FAS) has been estimated at between one and two per 1,000 live births.

The main issue is prevention, not diagnosis. In fact, labeling a child with that diagnosis can do more harm than good. Education at all levels of society is essential and cessation of drinking as soon as a pregnancy is suspected or confirmed could reduce or possibly prevent fetal damage. Some groups have even advocated incarceration for alcohol-addicted pregnant women, especially if they have had a previous child with FAS—most would view that approach as extreme and unacceptable. There are no known "safe" amounts of alcohol consumption and, as noted above, one single maternal binge episode at the wrong time could cause serious damage to the fetal brain.

Cocaine

Attempting to study the effects on the fetus of exposures to recreational drugs is extremely difficult because so often the exposures are to multiple drugs, including alcohol and cigarette smoke. In addition, usage is higher among mothers from lower socioeconomic groups where prenatal care and nutrition are more likely to be less than optimal. Reviews of multiple publications have shown no detectable increased risk of malformations in the offspring of well-documented cocaine users, with the possible exception of urinary tract anomalies. However, recent work has shown that cocaine-exposed infants do show higher rates of IUGR (24% versus 8%), head circumference below the 10th percentile (20% versus 5%), and neurological abnormalities including hypertonia, coarse tremor, and extensor leg posture. Of interest is the fact that the degree of damage increased significantly with increasing amounts of cocaine used by the mother. Narcotics do not appear to be teratogenic in humans but infants of, for example, heroin-dependent women, are at risk of neonatal withdrawal and sudden infant death.

Cigarettes

The association between cigarette smoking and low birth weight, with its increased risk of perinatal morbidity and mortality, is well known. In addition, there are increased risks for prematurity, miscarriages, and sudden infant death syndrome. Long-term studies are accumulating evidence for neurotoxicity affecting neurobehavioral development. Some of the toxic effects of cigarette smoke on the fetus could result from increased fetal concentrations of carboxyhemoglobin resulting from inhaled carbon monoxide getting into the fetal circulation; since carboxyhemoglobin binds oxygen more tightly than fetal or adult hemoglobin, there might be fetal tissue hypoxia and hence the interference with growth.

Occupational Exposures and Physical Agents

The most common calls to teratology information services about occupational exposures during pregnancy are regarding video display terminals (VDTs), organic solvents, and lead.

The **VDTs** do not emit radiation that can affect the fetus (proven by direct measurements and epidemiological studies of pregnant women), and there are no recognizable malformation syndromes attributable to any of the **organic solvents**.

Lead

Lead is certainly toxic to the developing fetal brain, just as it is to an adult brain; high levels in the maternal circulation can lead to high fetal blood levels, which are hazardous to fetal brain development and might even increase the risk of malformations, although no specific anomalies have been attributed to lead toxicity outside the CNS. Maternal exposures occur in, for example, the stained-glass industry, paint and battery manufacturing, and from moonshine whiskey. Maternal lead levels need to be assessed in terms of background lead levels in the community.

Radiation

Radiation is probably the most frequent cause of maternal anxiety from a physical agent during pregnancy. Studies have shown that fetal doses below 50 rads do not cause malformations (*diagnostic* radiation studies would rarely if ever expose a fetus to doses above 5 rads) and the post–atom bomb investigations in Hiroshima and Nagasaki failed to demonstrate an increased incidence of malformations among fetuses exposed in utero. *Therapeutic* radiation obviously is hazardous and the malformation attributed to radiation has been microcephaly. There is no evidence of risk from diagnostic radioisotopes.

Maternal Disease

Maternal Insulin-Dependent Diabetes Mellitus

Diabetes is unquestionably associated with an increased risk of fetal malformations of almost all types with anomalies of the heart and NTDs being most common, followed by skeletal, gastrointestinal (GI), and urinary tract anomalies. In addition, there is increased neonatal morbidity and mortality with prematurity, macrosomatia, respiratory distress, hypoglycemia, and other difficulties. The risk of all of these is greatly reduced by rigorous control of maternal glucose levels from preconception to delivery. The pregnancy must be managed as high risk and a team approach is ideal (family physician, obstetrician, and internist, with a pediatrician or neonatologist involved and ready to manage the newborn infant).

Maternal Phenylketonuria

Most individuals with PKU go off the rigorous diet in late childhood and a population of women running high levels of phenylalanine is now in the childbearing age group. It has been amply demonstrated that there is a marked increase in the incidence of liveborn infants with microcephaly and mental retardation, approaching 100%, among mothers with PKU! All women with known PKU should go back on the low-phenylalanine diet as teenagers to ensure that their phenylalanine levels are as close to normal as possible if and when conception occurs. Starting the diet early in a pregnancy might reduce the neurotoxic effect of phenylalanine and its metabolites but usually does not prevent it.

An additional and fortunately rare problem is the adult woman with undetected PKU: she is usually only mildly intellectually handicapped but with a distinctly increased blood phenylalanine level. All of her offspring will have varying degrees of microcephaly and mental handicap. Obviously, it is important to include a maternal blood phenylalanine level study in the investigation of neonatal or infantile microcephaly of unknown cause. PKU is discussed in more detail in chapter 5, "Newborn Screening."

LEARNING POINTS

Here is a list of the various human teratogens discussed in this chapter. Keep current by checking possible teratogens with your local teratogen service or the current literature on-line.

Maternal Infection

- Toxoplasmosis
- Rubella
- Cytomegalovirus
- Varicella
- Syphilis
- Herpes simplex

Maternal Drugs

- Chemotherapeutic agents. For example, alkylating agents and anti-metabolites
- Anticonvulsants. Hydantoin, trimethadione, valproate (none has been proven safe)
- Anticoagulants. Warfarin
- Sex steroids. Oral contraceptives (probably not teratogenic)
- Tranquilizers and antipsychosis agents. Carbamazepine, lithium, fluoxetine (Prozac)
- Vitamin A derivatives. Retinoic acid, tretinoin
- Antibiotics. Tetracyclines are not true teratogens

Recreational Drugs

- Cocaine
- Alcohol
- Cigarettes

Occupational Exposures and Physical Agents

- Organic solvents
- Lead
- Video display terminals
- Radiation

Maternal Disease

- Diabetes mellitus
- PKU

Further Reading

Kalow W. Pharmacogenetics in biological perspective. Pharmacol Rev 1997;49:369–79.
Koren G. Maternal-fetal toxicity. A clinician's guide. 3rd ed. New York: Marcel Decker, Inc.; 2001.
Polifka JE, Friedman JH. Clinical teratology: identifying teratogenic risks in humans. Clin Genet 1999;56:409–20.

Web Site

Organization of Teratology Information Services   <http://www.otispregnancy.org/>
Organization of Teratology Information Services (OTIS) offers a listing of services and centers in Canada and the United States, the latter, state by state. The organization also can be contacted by telephone at (888) 285-3410.

Pharmacogenetics: Pharmacogenomics

Clinical Scenario

The Smith family—mom, dad, and the two children, Sammy, age 8 years, and Sarah, age 11—set out for their annual summer month at the cottage. Sam, ordinarily a rather rambunctious youngster, was uncharacteristically quiet in the car and intermittently fell asleep. The parents noted that when they stopped for lunch, he appeared pale but not otherwise ill; he had no cough, runny nose, or other signs of a cold. As the afternoon wore on, he became increasingly pale and lethargic. Now alarmed, the family stopped at a small-town hospital emergency room. The ER physician found no abnormal physical signs other than pallor and lethargy. It was too late in the day for much of a laboratory work-up but the hemoglobin level was down to 70 g/L and the smear showed remarkable poikilocytosis with occasional spherocytes and many fragmented red cells. The white count and differential were normal. Acute hemolytic anemia was suspected and arrangements were made for transfer to a hospital in a larger community about an hour away. On arrival, the hemoglobin had fallen a bit further, and a reticulocyte count was markedly elevated. The sclerae were by then slightly yellow. Blood and urine were obtained for further study, and transfusion was ordered.

While the assigned physician was taking additional history and chatting with the family, a very friendly cleaning lady entered the room and overheard some of the story. After she had a brief discussion with the mother, she blurted out a diagnosis! It turned out that she was correct; although the transfusion was set up it never had to be given.

Now, we need some hypotheses. It seems reasonable to conclude that the original ER physician was correct: Sam had acute hemolytic anemia. This is not primarily a hematology exercise, but take a few moments to review and think about the possible causes of acute hemolytic anemia. There aren't very many. First you need to come up with the two possible sites of the pathogenesis and then some of the specific conditions.

Etiology of Acute Hemolytic Anemia

1. Extravascular (conditions due to defects extrinsic to the red cell)
   - **Hypersplenism**. Hypersplenism is seen in many diseases associated with reticuloendothelial hyperplasia. Since the pathogenetic process is sequestration of red cells, cell morphology is unchanged and there is splenomegaly. This is obviously not the case here.
   - **Autoimmune hemolytic anemia** The onset of autoimmune hemolytic anemia is usually abrupt, often there is splenomegaly, and there can be some red-cell morphological changes, such as spherocytosis and polychromatophilia. The hallmark is the presence of red-cell autoantibodies detectable by the Coombs' test (direct for antibodies on the red-cell membrane and indirect for antibodies free in the plasma). The most frequent cause is a drug reaction. This is a possibility.
   - **Infectious agents**. The hemolysis can result from the production by the organism of erythrotoxins (e.g., β-hemolytic streptococci) or by direct invasion of the red cell by the organism, as in malaria.
2. Intravascular (conditions intrinsic to the red cell)
   - Alterations of the red-cell membrane. Spherocytosis, elliptocytosis
   - Disorders of red-cell metabolism. The hereditary enzyme deficiencies, by far the most common being glucose-6-phosphate dehydrogenase (G6PD) deficiency
   - Hemoglobinopathies. The thalassemias, sickle cell disease, and so on.

Any ideas as to what's going on with Sammy Smith? The cleaning lady, an Italian woman, did what none of the doctors had gotten around to—she took a **family** history! As soon as she discovered that Sammy's mom was "Senora Taviani" and that her family came from a village in Sicily near hers, she guessed the diagnosis. Have you got it? Sure you have—"Il favismo!" Favism, alias primaquine sensitivity, alias G6PD deficiency.

What precipitated the hemolysis? Sammy hadn't been sick and was on no medications. However, the next-door neighbors at home were growing fava beans in their garden. They had dried and salted some, and had given Sammy some to taste the day before the Smiths left for their cottage. He loved them and ate several handfuls over the afternoon.

GLUCOSE-6-PHOSPHATE DEHYDROGENASE DEFICIENCY

History

Before looking into the issues relevant to pharmacogenetics in general, let's review the details of G6PD deficiency, the most common by far of the inherited enzyme deficiencies that affect the human red blood cell. In fact, it is probably the first example of a pharmacogenetic disorder to be described—Pythagoras, in southern Italy about 500 BC, recognized that some individuals who ate fava beans became ill, while others could enjoy them with no adverse effects. It wasn't until the late 1940s that William Boyd, an immunochemist from Boston University, noted that the British, in contrast to Mediterranean populations, never developed hemolytic anemia on ingestion of fava beans and suggested a genetic difference as the probable explanation. In the Pacific theater prior to and during World War II, scientists from the University of Chicago observed that about 10% of black American soldiers and, rarely, some of the white soldiers, developed hemolytic anemia of varying severity when given conventional doses of a then-new antimalarial drug, primaquine. In 1956, further studies showed that the susceptible individuals' red cells were G6PD deficient and in 1958, Barton Childs and colleagues at Johns Hopkins University showed that the enzyme defect is inherited as an X-linked trait.

Biochemistry

Affected individuals, usually males, are normal until given one of several drugs (Table 9–1) or uncooked fava beans. The drugs' common characteristic is that they are all oxidizing agents. The causative constituent of fava beans is still not clear, although a pyrimidine aglycone has been strongly implicated. Cooking the beans destroys their hemolytic capacity. Even the mechanisms responsible for the oxidative hemolysis are far from clear. Curiously, the red cell of the deficient person as it enters the circulation usually has a normal or at least an adequate amount of G6PD, but the structural defect almost always renders the molecule unstable and the levels rapidly fall. The deficiency of G6PD activity destabilizes the erythrocyte membrane and hence the hemolysis. Only the older red cells are susceptible to hemolysis and they are rapidly destroyed following ingestion of one of the drugs or fava beans. The hemolysis, therefore, is self-limited and the resulting reticulocytosis will usually compensate for the hemolysis. Hemoglobin levels return to near normal within a few days even if the drug is continued or the individual continues to eat fava beans.

Literally hundreds of G6PD variants have been found in deficient individuals around the world but in general, the mutant alleles found commonly in black populations leave the affected males with a relatively milder

Table 9–1
Agents that Can Cause Hemolysis in G6PD-Deficient People

Antimalarial drugs
- primaquine
- pamaquine
- pentaquine
- chloroquine

Sulfonamides

Nitrofurans (Furadantin)

Phenacetin (acetominophen, acetanilid)

Naphthalene

Vitamin K derivatives

Fava beans

Acetylsalicylic acid

Probenecid (Benemid)

hemolytic anemia than white individuals from the various Mediterranean populations.

Genetics and Epidemiology

As would be expected for an X-linked trait, the majority of affected individuals are male. However, since the overall frequency among, for example, black males is 10%, homozygous G6PD-deficient females are not all that uncommon.

How common **is** the homozygous female? That's easy! Did you all get one in 100 for black females? And why is that? Well, if one in 10 black males has an X chromosome with a deficiency gene, then the prevalence of the deficiency alleles in that population is obviously one in 10. Thus, the chance of a female having a deficiency allele twice is $1/10 \times 1/10$.

Carriers or heterozygotes also have reduced levels of G6PD in their red cells, but certainly among blacks, the frequency of clinically evident hemolysis is small. A proportion of Mediterranean carrier females is susceptible to hemolysis but as expected, the severity is generally less than for affected males.

Worldwide, G6PD deficiency is the most common enzyme disorder of humans. In some villages in Sardinia, for example, close to 70% of males were found to be G6PD deficient. It is a globally important cause of neonatal jaundice and can lead to life-threatening hemolytic crises both in childhood and the adult years through interaction with drugs and fava beans in the diet.

G6PD deficiency is one of the intrinsic red-cell disorders that has been selected for survival by the malaria parasite, the others being thalassemia and sickle cell disease. It has been shown experimentally that the malarial parasite requires host cell G6PD for its own survival and replication, and without a relatively normal amount of it, the parasite dies rather than the host. Since the mortality rate for favism is low, and the mortality rate for falciparum malaria is high (infant mortality rates in some parts of Sardinia after World War II, following deliberate flooding of some coastal areas by departing German troops, approached 50%), the protective effect of the enzyme deficiency is significant. In addition, there could be a small protective effect for the heterozygous female. The world distribution map of G6PD deficiency overlays very neatly onto the map for the distribution of falciparum malaria (Figure 9–1, A and B) and it includes the Mediterranean area, parts of Africa, the Middle East, India, and southern Asia.

Clinical Presentation

The severity of the hemolysis depends on the drug and the dose, as well as the specific mutant allele the person inherited. Clinical manifestations include pallor, irritability, abdominal and back pain (renal colic), red urine caused by hemoglobinuria, and mild jaundice appearing within 72 hours of ingestion. The episodes are usually self-limited and last about 1 week whether or not the precipitating agent is continued. Uncommonly, there can be a fulminating hemolysis with death due to acute anemia.

In the newborn with any one of the several mutations seen mainly in the white population, for example, people of Mediterranean origin, the deficiency is a contributing cause of increased hyperbilirubinemia, which if untreated can lead to kernicterus with resulting brain damage.

The diagnosis depends on the following:

- History. The ethnic or national/geographical origin of the patient and the ingestion of one of the known oxidative drugs or fava beans
- Laboratory data consistent with drug-induced hemolytic anemia
- Demonstration of G6PD deficiency or a specific mutant G6PD allele

Measurement of enzyme activity during an episode of hemolysis might cause you to miss the diagnosis. Why? Remember, the hemolysis and drop in hemoglobin level causes reticulocytosis and the reticulocytes enter the circulation with usually normal levels of G6PD.

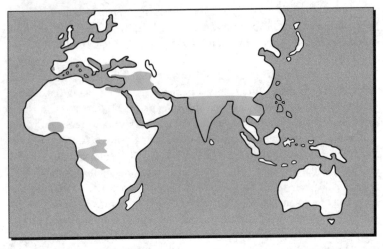

A

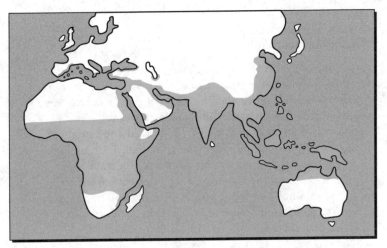

B

Figure 9–1 World distribution of *A*, G6PD deficiency and *B*, falciparum malaria.

Management

Stopping the drug will put an end to further hemolysis and obviously is appropriate even though the course of the illness is usually self-limiting. Curiously, people who know they suffer from favism often live in relatively poor areas where the beans are a staple portion of their diet; they know that at the beginning of the fava bean season, they will develop the clinical signs but they put up with them knowing they will soon abate. Fortunately, few will die.

With patients like Sammy, monitoring the hemoglobin is sufficient, and most of the time it will not be necessary to transfuse. Newborn infants with hyperbilirubinemia due to G6PD deficiency are treated in the usual way with phototherapy and, if necessary, exchange transfusion.

PHARMACOGENETICS

The term pharmacogenetics is defined as the study of variability in drug response as a result of heredity. Another term has been introduced recently —**pharmacogenomics**, the field that emphasizes the development of novel drugs based on newly discovered genes. The two terms can be used practically interchangeably.

Why is the subject considered to be of sufficient importance to be included in the PDQ series? Although G6PD deficiency is common, the rest of the *specific* disorders mentioned below are rare. The main issue, however, is adverse drug reaction (ADR), which in the United States accounts for an astonishing 6% to 7% of admissions to hospital. In 1994, for example, 106,000 *fatal* ADRs were reported. Obviously, not all ADRs are due to toxicity secondary to inherited variation in the way drugs are absorbed and metabolized, but a very high proportion are, as the following discussion will demonstrate.

Think for a moment about what happens when a drug is taken. First, it has to get absorbed into the blood either orally or by injection (Figure 9–2). There are four basic processes: uptake, binding and distribution, metabolism, and excretion. For the first step, a drug has to find its way into the bloodstream. Some drugs will diffuse passively; others will be actively transported by specific transport proteins. Wherever there are proteins, inevitably there will be genetic variation; some patients will be rapid transporters of certain drugs, some will be slow, and most of the time there will be a multitude of variants in between. In addition, some transporters will bind their drug molecule tightly; others lightly, all because of variations in binding sites that are genetically determined. Proteolytic enzymes in the blood can interfere with the effective dose of a drug, and some drugs or their drug-transporter complex can trigger an immune response. Within a cell, drugs can be oxygenated to an active form or conjugated and then transported to a target organelle or to the nucleus. Although most drugs are metabolized and excreted rapidly, some are sequestered in certain tissues; the Accutane group described in the previous chapter comes to mind. They are absorbed into fat and can be slowly released over several days to weeks. Figure 9–2 depicts and summarizes many of the steps that a drug must take to get from the mouth or needle to its final target within a specific cell in a specific tissue.

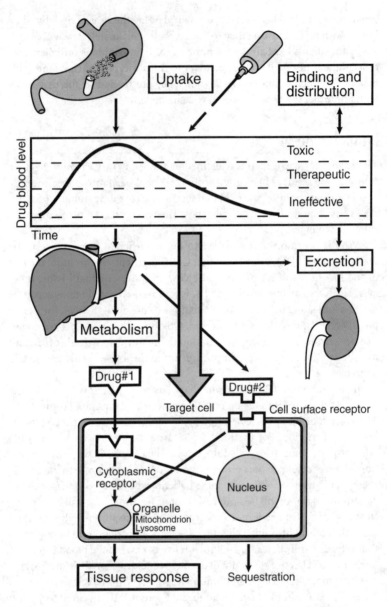

Figure 9–2 Schematic depiction of pathways from drug administration to tissue response.

During the 1970s, the US government "declared war" on sickle cell disease as part of a somewhat misguided effort to improve medical services to the black community. Federal funding was provided specifically for research and for clinics to support free screening of adults for carrier status. The intent was to identify carrier parents at risk of having homozygous affected offspring: counseling, data on early detection of affected infants, and prenatal diagnosis were to be provided. Unfortunately, education and counseling facilities were grossly inadequate and inevitably, being a heterozygote was frequently interpreted as having a disease. In 1979 six black men were expelled from the Air Force Academy in Colorado Springs because they had been screened and found to be sickle cell disease carriers. The grounds for dismissal: their health might be endangered by the strain of rigorous training at the academy's altitude of about 7,000 feet. Furthermore, some airlines required carrier screening for black applicants for flight attendant training and rejected those who tested positive. Curiously, pilots were not required to have the carrier test. There is no valid evidence that carriers are at increased risk during exertion at high altitudes and I dare say that should an aircraft depressurize at 30,000 feet, sickle cell carriers would be in no greater trouble than noncarriers!

Obviously, the above and the following examples go a bit beyond the strict definition of "pharmacogenetics" (hypoxia is hardly a drug, nor are beryllium and other air pollutants), but they are included in this section because of the impact that screening in the workplace is already having and will unquestionably continue to have. The general concept of an underlying variant with no effect other than causing a predisposition to an environmental agent is identical. Let's look briefly at industrial pollutants from a genetic point of view.

Beryllium

Excessive quantities of beryllium in the dust and fumes emitted from power plants fueled by burning coal can raise beryllium concentrations in the atmosphere by greater than 100-fold as compared to levels found in nonindustrial locales. Occupational beryllium disease, **berylliosis**, also occurs in high-technology industries such as ceramics manufacturing, electronics, dental alloy preparation, and nuclear weapons manufacturing.

Berylliosis, or **chronic beryllium disease** (CBD), is serious with an insidious onset, sometimes over many years. It begins with shortness of breath on exertion and cough, both of which progressively worsen. Burning chest pain, shortness of breath even at rest, anorexia, weight loss, and right heart failure can ensue and result in early death. The picture is that of chronic obstructive respiratory disease with progressive pulmonary fibrosis. There is also a dermatological form of berylliosis manifesting as poor wound healing and a papular rash often with wart-like bumps on palms, fingers, and forearms. The pathogenesis is immunological, requiring initial exposure of skin or inhalation for sensitization.

Approximately 5% of exposed individuals develop the disease. Why not everyone? The complete answer to that question is not yet in. Possibly anyone can develop it after sufficient exposure. However, HLA-DPβ1-Glu69 is a genetic marker for susceptibility. Studies have shown that up to 97% of CBD patients have the Glu69 marker, but 30% to 45% of beryllium-exposed *unaffected* individuals also carry the same marker. Homozygotes are much more susceptible to CBD than are heterozygotes. Clearly, the presence of Glu69 is not the sole genetic factor underlying the susceptibility for CBD.

Studies in progress include one of the major producers and suppliers of beryllium for industrial use. Prospective employees are being given the opportunity to voluntarily undergo screening for the Glu69 marker and if positive, counseling regarding risk and options are being provided. The options are rejection of the job or monitoring for early signs of illness. With early diagnosis and prompt institution of steroid or other immunosuppressive therapy, the development of CBD is prevented or significantly slowed.

α_1-Antitrypsin Deficiency

α_1-Antitrypsin (α_1-AT) deficiency is an inherited enzyme deficiency that causes an increased risk of liver disease in children and an increased risk of chronic obstructive lung disease in adults. It is one of the most common inherited anomalies of the white population with a prevalence of between one in 7,000 to one in 2,000.

The probable pathogenesis is inadequate inactivation of enzymes with trypsin-like activity in the liver and lung resulting in autodestruction with inflammation and subsequent fibrosis. Several alleles of α_1-AT cause varying degrees of deficiency in both the homozygous and heterozygous states (see "Further Reading" for more data). Again, homozygotes are at highest risk of early-onset emphysema: cigarette smoking greatly increases the risk.

Also in the 1970s, Dow Chemical started testing prospective employees for α_1-AT deficiency. The rationale was that if pollutants in cigarette smoke hastened the onset of chronic obstructive lung disease, industrial pollutants might do the same. There was and still is no evidence that this is the case. Altruistically, the claim was that the industry was trying to protect the genetically susceptible by testing and then either not hiring those found to be deficient or employing them in areas of low pollution, generally in lower-paying jobs outside the mines and processing plants. Practically, the industry might have been attempting to protect itself from the expense of training personnel only to have them become sick and less productive in a relatively short time. In addition, the possibility of individual or class action lawsuits loomed. However, the union viewed the testing as an unfair labor practice and maintained that the onus should be on the industry to make the workplace safe for everyone, regardless of their α_1-AT status. Testing was soon stopped by the company, which claimed that the program didn't supply useful information.

LEARNING POINTS

- The enormous variability in response to and susceptibility to toxic effects of drugs and environmental pollutants has a major genetic component.
- The mutant alleles, in general and in an evolutionary sense, have nothing to do with drug metabolism. They arose spontaneously and those that achieved polymorphism status (a frequency greater than 1%) were presumably established in various human populations by natural selection in relation to steps in *normal* intermediary metabolism.
- With the exception of G6PD deficiency, the selective agents are unknown.
- The establishment of G6PD deficiency at such high frequencies in certain populations illustrates the rapidity with which selection can occur if the selective force is sufficiently potent.
- In most cases, the mutant alleles cause no clinical manifestations unless or until there is some external challenge.
- G6PD deficiency is a common X-linked condition that must be kept in mind by all physicians when prescribing any of the drugs listed in Table 9–1 or when a patient, especially a male, presents with unexplained intravascular hemolytic anemia.
- The importance of being aware of principles of pharmacogenetics is further exemplified by (1) the replacement of the almost ubiquitously used succinylcholine by nonpolarizing muscle relaxants safe for all individuals, whether pseudocholinesterase deficient or not; and (2) an awareness of the possibility of malignant hyperthermia by anesthetists and the availability of the antidote, dantrolene, in virtually all operating rooms.
- The implications of screening for genetic predispositions in the workplace, including ethical and insurance issues, privacy, and the need for well thought out facilities for education and counseling, must be kept firmly in mind.

Further Reading

Childs B, Zinkham WH, Browne EA, et al. A genetic study of a defect in glutathione metabolism of the erythrocyte. Bull Johns Hopkins *Hosp* 1958;1-2:21–37.

Evans DAP, Manley KA, McKusick VA. Genetic control of isoniazid metabolism in man. BMJ 1960;2:485–91.

Harris H. Garrod's inborn errors of metabolism. London: Oxford University Press; 1963.

Nebert DW. Pharmacogenetics and pharmacogenomics: why is this relevant to the clinical geneticist? Clin Genet 1999;56:247–58.

Snyder LH. Studies in human inheritance. IX. The inheritance of taste deficiency in man. Ohio J Sci 1932;32:436–68.

Weber WW. Pharmacogenetics. New York: Oxford University Press; 1997.

Neurodegenerative Diseases

Clinical Scenario

One of your patients, George Davis, a 34-year-old man, accompanies his mother, Doris, to see you. She is a 55-year-old woman whose behavior has become an increasing worry for the family. As far back as the children can remember, Mother always liked her vodka and tonic at the end of the day; she probably had one before Dad got home from work, and always had another one or two with him. It was not unusual for her to be a bit tipsy in the evening but never really drunk. Her husband died about 1 year ago of a heart attack and ever since, Doris had become more and more unusual. The family noticed that her speech was slurred and she was becoming increasingly clumsy, dropping things such as kitchen utensils and dishes with increasing frequency. She was also becoming quite forgetful and, as George explained, just last week he and his wife had made a date to take her out for dinner; when they arrived to pick her up, she was not ready and then got quite agitated, insisting that the dinner date was for the following evening.

In addition, George mentioned that his mother's gait was becoming abnormal—she often appeared as if she had had too much to drink. At first, everyone thought that perhaps she was having a few extra drinks in the process of grieving for her recently deceased husband, but she denied this vehemently, claiming that she'd hardly drunk at all since she had no one to drink with any more. In fact, one of the observations that precipitated this visit to the doctor was George's discovery that a special bottle of vodka he'd given his mother as a gift about 6 months previously had not been opened.

The history was entirely negative. Doris had never been seriously ill and had never been admitted to hospital except for the deliveries of her three children.

The family history indicated that Doris was an only child. She and her husband emigrated from Czechoslovakia just prior to World War II. Her father, a heavy smoker, died of lung cancer at age 42. Little was known of his family but he had mentioned over the years that he'd had a sister who never married and who was in an institution as an adult—he didn't know what the problem was but he remembered her as being normal as a child and young adult; she died while in that institution and apparently was severely disabled by that time. Doris's mother was an 80-year-old woman and remarkably healthy; she emigrated to North America with the family. Her siblings and their children stayed in Czechoslovakia and all perished in the Holocaust. George has two siblings, a brother age 30 and a sister age 25. Both are in good health and are single. George has two children, both boys, ages 12 and 10.

On physical examination, Doris was fidgety, quite unable to sit still. Again, she denied drinking at all, and, indeed, there was no odor of alcohol on her breath. Mentally she was fairly alert but somewhat disoriented with regard to time and space—she was unsure of which day of the week it was and couldn't recall very accurately what she had done for the two or three days prior to this visit to the office. Her speech was slightly slurred. She had no abnormal eye movements but her gait was wide-based and mildly ataxic. There was generalized hyperreflexia.

INTRODUCTION

What are your hypotheses at this point?

Although the family history is unclear (see "Mode of Inheritance" below), the combination of progressive motor and cognitive disturbances have to put Huntington's disease at the top of your list, though the dysarthria and ataxia raise the possibility of one of the cerebellar ataxias. Other types of presenile dementias are rare and are not usually associated with neurological signs. The fidgeting and inability to sit still are early signs of chorea—other causes of chorea need to be considered, including thyrotoxicosis, cerebellar disease, and benign hereditary chorea. A more detailed differential diagnosis is given below.

What is your next step?

It is probably not a good idea to run a list of possible diagnoses by the family at this point, although you will have to let them know that the signs and symptoms could indicate a neurological condition. You could suggest that the family history is something that needs to be taken into consideration. But before any details are discussed, it would be best to do the diagnostic deoxyribonucleic acid (DNA) test for the relatively common condition known as Huntington's disease.

This creates a decision point: you could refer the patient and her family now to a neurological center, where a multidisciplinary team is organized

to work with families with possible Huntington's disease and related neurodegenerative disorders, or you could order the molecular test yourself
and then refer the patient and her family.

HUNTINGTON'S DISEASE

This is a good time to review briefly the features of Huntington's disease.

Clinical Manifestations

Huntington's disease is characterized by progressive motor, cognitive, and
psychiatric deterioration. The average age of onset is between 35 and
45 years. However, approximately 25% of cases have their onset in the
50s or even later and very rarely, manifestations can begin in childhood,
as early as age 10 years. Usually the early signs include subtle changes in
coordination, minor involuntary movements, clumsiness, memory loss,
especially in planning day-to-day activities, and often variable degrees
of depression or irritability. Later, choreiform movements become more
obvious with increasing difficulty with voluntary activity, worsening
dysarthria, and dysphagia. (Chorea is an involuntary movement disorder
with nonrepetitive and nonperiodic jerking of limbs, face, or trunk present
continuously during the waking hours; it cannot be suppressed voluntarily
and it is made worse by stress. Huntington's disease used to be called Huntington's chorea—more than 90% of patients develop chorea/choreiform
movements.)

With advancing duration of the disease, involuntary movements worsen,
often with development of hypokinesia, rigidities, and dystonia. In addition, fine and gross motor control is progressively impeded.

Oculomotor disturbances tend to occur early and then worsen over
time. There could be problems with gaze fixation and abnormally jerky eye
movements when changing focus.

Decreasing cognitive abilities are inevitable and eventually there are
personality changes that can advance to frank psychosis.

Gradually the patient becomes more and more dependent on caregivers,
eventually becoming totally helpless. To make matters worse, most affected
individuals show intermittent bursts of aggressive behavior and social dis-
inhibition. The average age at death is 54 to 55 years.

Prevalence

The prevalence of Huntington's disease is between three and seven per
100,000 in populations of western European descent, achieving a maximum
prevalence of more than 15 per 100,000 in some areas where the people are

of western European origin. It is less common in east Asian countries, Scandinavia, and among African blacks.

Diagnosis

Diagnosis depends on recognition of the characteristic clinical presentation and then confirmation of diagnosis through DNA testing. Pathologically, there is generalized brain atrophy, especially involving the caudate nuclei and the putamen. Later there is compensatory dilatation of the ventricles, especially in the frontal lobes (the anterior horns of the lateral ventricles), where loss of substance of the caudate nuclei causes concavity of the floor of the ventricles, leading to what is commonly referred to as **box car ventricles**, as seen on computed tomography (CT) or magnetic resonance imaging (MRI) scans. Since the advent of molecular diagnosis, brain imaging studies are no longer indicated— earlier on they are usually negative and later, they are hardly needed.

Differential Diagnosis

Huntington's disease is one of the presenile dementias and the possible etiological considerations include the classic categories of disease: intoxicant, infectious, vascular, neoplastic, genetic, and traumatic. Trauma, other than causing chronic subdural hematoma (see "Neoplastic" below) is unlikely to lead to Huntington's disease manifestations.

Intoxicant

As in this case, chronic alcohol use must be kept in mind, along with the possibility of prescription drug overdose or incompatibility (the latter is occurring with increased frequency as multiple physicians looking after especially elderly patients prescribe antidepressant drugs without knowing that the patient is taking one or even several already—some combinations can have more than additive effects!). Abuse of hallucinogenic drugs is another possibility.

Infection

Many of the chronic infectious diseases of the brain (bacterial, fungal, and viral) can present with dementia, including AIDS and Creutzfeldt-Jakob disease. The movement disorder of the latter is myoclonus, and it usually appears with the first 6 months of the illness.

Vascular

Hypertension and atherosclerosis can cause multiple cerebral infarcts and lead to dementia, as can emboli from the heart or elsewhere. Chronic heart disease with cerebral ischemia or hypoxia is also on the list.

Neoplastic

Both benign and malignant tumors of the brain, as well as chronic subdural hematomas, can cause dementia with or without neurological signs. Obstructive hydrocephalus and the rare but much talked about **normal pressure hydrocephalus** are causes of dementia and gait disturbances.

Genetic

Alzheimer's and Parkinson's disease should not cause confusion for long. The very rare Pick's disease mimics Huntington's disease; it is distinguishable by neuroimaging: atrophy affects mainly the frontal and temporal lobes.

Management

Management of Huntington's disease is symptomatic. The chorea can be decreased with the neuroleptic agents and antiparkinson drugs might decrease the hypokinesia and rigidity. Psychiatric symptoms, such as depression and aggression, might respond to psychotropic drugs. The main management issue is support for the family, which might consist of making sure that they are aware of the Huntington's Disease Association and of community resources, including home nursing visits, and other community support systems.

Mode of Inheritance

Huntington's disease is inherited as an autosomal dominant trait. Most affected individuals have an affected parent. A negative family history can result from a variety of phenomena:

- Spontaneous mutation. Since the discovery of the actual causative mutation, new mutations have been confirmed in as many as a quarter of the cases (see further reading).
- The vagaries of the family history. This is an issue in the clinical scenario, where the possibly affected parent died of an unrelated cause (a heart attack) before the expected age of onset. The history of the father's sister having a probable adult-onset degenerative disease is certainly compatible with a diagnosis of Huntington's disease.
- Decreased penetrance (see below).

Historical Review of the Search for the Huntington's Gene

In 1983, tight linkage was found with a DNA marker on the short arm of chromosome 4. This discovery marked the beginning of predictive testing for asymptomatic family members, and although the linkage was indeed close, errors due to crossovers did, of course, occur.

It took 10 more years to find the actual mutation and it turned out to be an expansion of a CAG/polyglutamine tract in exon one. Patients with Huntington's disease have 36 to 121 repeats, with a mean of 40.

- Patients with adult-onset illness usually have 40 to 55 repeats, whereas juvenile-onset cases usually have more than 50, and in almost all juvenile cases, the expanded allele is inherited from the father.
- There is an inverse relationship between the CAG repeat length and the age of onset of the disease.
- Penetrance in the 36 to 41 repeat range is reduced.
- The product of the *HD* gene has been named *huntingtin*. Since CAG codes for glutamine, the uninterrupted stretch of CAG repeats results in a polyglutamine insertion. The actual defect, that is, the pathogenesis and the reason for the long delay between conception and any clinical manifestation, are not known. One suggestion in relation to the pathogenesis is that protein–protein interactions mediated by polyglutamine tracts might simply result in insoluble and toxic precipitates.
- The gene locus is 4p16. CAG repeat lengths are highly variable in the normal population at 10 to 35 with a mean of 18; 15 to 20 repeats are the most common number in the normal population.
- An interesting point is that homozygotes for Huntington's disease are no more severely affected than heterozygotes, which is a distinctly unusual phenomenon. For example, the relatively rare homozygotes in most other dominant conditions that we know about are much more severely affected than the heterozygotes. Achondroplasia is a good example (see chapter 7, "Bone Dysplasias and Short Stature").
- The intermediate allele (27 to 35 repeats) or the reduced-penetrance allele (36 to 41 repeats) in an asymptomatic individual or in a person with a new mutation will not expand when transmitted by the mother, but there's a 2% to 3% chance of expansion into the disease range if transmitted by the father.

It is time to pause again to think about a major, relatively recently discovered, basic principle of genetics that flies in the face of what we learned from Mendel's experiments.

- Which of Mendel's laws is violated by the CAG expansion data in families?
- What is the term we use for the worsening of a condition (earlier age of onset and more severe clinical consequences) as it is passed down from parent to offspring within a family?
- Can you name another condition in which this phenomenon occurs?

The answers to these questions and a brief discussion are included in chapter 1 under "Exceptions to Mendelian Inheritance."

Clinical Scenario Continued

After a careful and detailed discussion with you, George and his mother decide to go ahead with the Huntington's gene expansion test for Doris. As you expected, it comes back positive—her expansion consists of 42 repeats. At the suggestion of the gene testing laboratory and with your enthusiastic agreement, the test result is to be given and discussed at the Medical Center in the Genetics Counseling Clinic. The geneticist and genetic counselor invite you to attend and you make time to do so. Naturally, the news was devastating for both George and Doris as the reality of an untreatable degenerative disease hit them, along with the issues pertinent to the genetics. The rest of the family would have to be informed and make decisions about testing for themselves and be told the implications for the children they might wish to have in the future.

Presymptomatic Testing

Testing of asymptomatic at-risk individuals for Huntington's disease has been available for more than a decade and has raised a large number of serious counseling and other issues. Predictive testing must involve pretest interviews in which the reasons for requesting the test, the individual's knowledge of the disease, the possible impact of either a positive or a negative test result, and the individual's neurological and psychological functioning are assessed. Posttest follow-ups are also essential no matter what the result of the test. Obviously, the discovery that one has the gene and will eventually and inevitably develop the disease manifestations will have a negative effect on most individuals who receive that information, but perhaps surprisingly, about 10% of those with decreased risk have serious difficulties adapting to their new status. This phenomenon of a negative response to good news is not uncommon and is often referred to as the **Holocaust syndrome**—guilt feelings found among survivors who wonder why they were spared and their relatives died.

Here's another very sensitive scenario. Consider a woman in the childbearing age group who is at risk (one in four) because of an affected grandparent but whose at-risk mother does not wish to know her status. Suppose the daughter is tested and does the right thing; that is, she does not give her mother her result, but, when pregnant, has amniocentesis.

It has been interesting to note, in view of the above, that overall, the demand for testing of at-risk asymptomatic adults has been lower than expected from the studies conducted before the availability of direct testing.

Requests from parents for testing at-risk children require sensitive and understanding counseling. The international consensus is that asymptomatic children should not have testing for a wide variety of reasons, including the possibility of stigmatization within the family and in other social settings. The results could have serious educational and career implications within a family. For example, suppose there are two siblings, one of whom tests positive and the other, negative. Would both be given equal opportunities for further education, especially if there were limited resources within that family?

If testing of a child becomes an issue in a family for whatever reason, the child himself or herself should be a major participant in arriving at a decision. That, of course, means that the child needs to be old enough and mature enough to understand all the implications; obviously, the appropriate age will vary from individual to individual. These issues are covered in detail on the American Society of Human Genetics Web site (<www.faseb.org/genetics/ashg/ashgmenu.htm>)—click on "Society Policy Statements and Reports" and then on "Points to Consider: Ethical, Legal, and Psychosocial Implications of Genetic Testing in Children and Adolescents."

Prenatal testing is technically available and highly accurate, as long as the mutant gene has been detected in a given family, but termination of a pregnancy for a disease with an average age of onset between 40 and 50 years raises many ethical issues.

Predictive testing also raises the serious issues of negative effects with regard to employment and life insurance, should such information fall into the hands of third parties.

GENE TESTING FOR THE HEREDITARY ATAXIAS

Had the test for Huntington's disease been negative in the clinical scenario, one of the groups of conditions that would have had to be excluded is the adult-onset hereditary ataxias. The likelihood is small—the majority are autosomal dominant disorders and ought to have a positive family history. However, the same factors that could distort the family histories in Huntington's disease could occur in this group as well. In addition, movement disorders are uncommon in these ataxias. Curiously, most, like Huntington's disease, are due to trinucleotide repeats.

One of the rare autosomal recessive ataxias, Friedreich's ataxia, is usually looked on as a childhood-onset disease, but with the availability of DNA testing, patients are being found with adult-onset forms. As is the case for many of the trinucleotide repeat disorders, in Friedreich's ataxia there is a correlation between the size of the repeat (in this disease, a GAA triplet repeat) and the clinical consequences: individuals with shorter repeats tend to be among the milder cases and have later ages of onset. It is important to note that as a general rule, when a specific biochemical or molecular defect is found as the cause for various genetic diseases, this knowledge soon contributes to the uncovering of much more clinical variability than had been described previously.

An up-to-date overview of the hereditary ataxias is presented on the GeneClinics Web site (<www.geneclinics.org/>) and the GeneTests Web site (<http://www.genetests.org/>). Search using "ataxia."

LEARNING POINTS

Huntington's disease, a relatively uncommon neurodegenerative disorder, is discussed here primarily to exemplify the problems of presymptomatic genetic disease testing.

- Prevalence ranges from one to 15 per 100,000 in populations mainly of western European origin
- Clinical manifestations. Progressive motor, cognitive, and psychiatric deterioration
- Age of onset. 35 to 40 years, with a downhill course to total incapacitation and death over 10 to 15 years from time of diagnosis
- Genetics. Inherited as an autosomal dominant trait; the gene locus is 4p16, the molecular defect is a trinucleotide repeat, and, at least for paternal transmission of the mutant allele, there is genetic "anticipation"
- Problems with presymptomatic testing. Psychosocial impact on at-risk individuals of *both* negative and positive results; ethics of testing under-age children; issues pertaining to prenatal diagnosis; effects on third parties (issues of confidentiality), including other family members, employers, and insurance companies

Further Reading

ACMG/ASHG Huntington Disease Genetic Testing Working Group. Laboratory guidelines for Huntington disease genetic testing. Am J Hum Genet 1998;62: 1243–7.

Almqvist EW, Elterman DS, MacLeod PM, et al. High incidence rate and absent family histories in one quarter of patients newly diagnosed with Huntington disease in British Columbia. Clin Genet 2001;60:198–205.

Huntington Disease Collaborative Research Group. A novel gene containing a trinucleotide repeat that is expanded and unstable on Huntington's disease chromosomes. Cell 1993;72:971–83.

Kolata G. Genetic screening raises questions for employers and insurers. Science 1986;232:317–9.

Web Sites

GeneClinics and GeneTests Web sites, under Huntington disease and ataxia:
<http://www.geneclinics.org/>
<http://www.genetests.org/>

Glossary

Amniotic bands Possibly as a result of tears in the amnion, amniotic strands float out into the amniotic sac and encircle fetal parts, most often the distal limbs. The result can be a constriction ring (see Figure 3–4), with or without impaired growth distally, or even amputation distal to the constriction. Rarely, amniotic bands can cause severe fetal distortion with asymmetric clefts of the face and cranium and what amounts to extrophies of chest and abdominal contents. Familial cases are extremely unusual.

Aneuploidy Having a chromosome number that is not an exact multiple of the haploid number characteristic of the species; for example, trisomy in humans is 47 chromosomes; tetrasomy is 48 chromosomes.

Angelman's syndrome A neurological disease characterized by severe mental retardation, microcephaly, absent speech, seizures, and a movement disorder that includes a broadly based jerky gait with arms flexed in abduction. The gait, along with a generally cheerful disposition and bursts of inappropriate laughter, led to its original designation as the "happy puppet syndrome." The cause is a chromsome 15q11–q13 maternally derived deletion or uncommonly, uniparental disomy. Compare with Prader-Willi syndrome.

Anticipation In the genetic sense, the phenomenon whereby some medical genetic conditions show earlier ages of onset and increasing severity of manifestations as the causative gene expands during passage from generation to generation. See chapter 1.

Beckwith-Wiedemann syndrome One of the "overgrowth" conditions characterized by high birth weight, often with asymmetry, macroglossia, and umbilical hernia or omphalocele. As part of the macrosomia, there is hyperplasia of the islets of Langerhans with resulting hyperinsulinemia and hypoglycemia; the low blood sugar is usually transient, but it can result in seizures and permanent brain damage. Beckwith-Wiedemann syndrome is one of the anomalies associated with imprinting, as discussed in chapter 1.

Cleidocranial dysostosis   An autosomal dominant condition characterized by hypoplasia to complete absence of the clavicles, delayed ossification of cranial sutures, large and late-closing anterior fontanelle, and delayed eruption of teeth.

Coffin-Lowry syndrome   An X-linked dominant clinical entity in which affected males are severely mentally retarded, have a characteristic coarse facial appearance with thick lips, and have typical large, soft hands with puffy, tapering fingers. Milder manifestations occur frequently in the heterozygous females, most of whom have normal to near-normal intellect.

Diploid   Having the chromosome number of the normal somatic cell; that is, with a pair of each of the chromosomes.

Ear creases   Seen in most newborns with Beckwith-Wiedemann syndrome (see Figure 3–14). Sometimes they are on the medial aspect of the lobe.

Embryo   The early or developing stage of any organism; in humans, the period from 1 week through 8 weeks after conception.

Epicanthal fold   Figure 3–10 shows the typical epicanthal fold seen in Down syndrome, other chromosome anomalies, and several other conditions not associated with chromosome defects.

Expressivity   The extent to which a trait is manifest; that is, the trait can vary in expression from mild to severe. Compare with penetrance.

Fanconi's anemia   An autosomal recessive syndrome characterized by unilateral hypoplasia or aplasia of the radial side of an upper limb (sometimes with total absence of the thumb) and occasionally microcephaly with developmental delay. Bone marrow hypoplasia is inevitable in childhood with eventual pancytopenia and a predisposition to leukemia and other malignancies.

Fetus   The developing offspring in the human uterus from the end of the second month of gestation. The fetus becomes an infant when it is completely outside the body of the mother.

Founder effect   High prevalence of a mutant gene in a population founded by a small group where one or more were carriers of that mutant gene, i.e., a mutant gene can achieve high prevalence without any selective advantage.

Genetic counseling   "A communication process which deals with the human problems associated with the occurrence or risk of occurrence of a genetic disorder in a family. This process involves an attempt by one or more appropriately trained persons to help the individual or family to: (1) comprehend the medical facts including the diagnosis, probable course of the disorder, and the available management, (2) appreciate the way heredity contributes to the disorder and the risk of recurrence in specified relatives, (3) understand the alternatives for dealing with the risk of recurrence, (4) choose a course of action which seems to them appropriate in view of their risk, their family goals, and their ethical and religious standards and act in accordance with that decision, and (5) to make the best possible adjustment to the disorder in an affected family member and/or to the risk of recurrence of that disorder" (as proposed by a committee of the American Society of Human Genetics, 1975).

Genotype   The genetic constitution of an individual, usually in reference to the alleles present at a specific genetic locus.

Haploid   Having the chromosome number of the normal gamete with only one member of each chromosome pair.

Hemizygote   A term that applies to the genotype of an individual with only one representative of a chromosome or a segment of a chromosome; used primarily in reference to a male with a variant or mutant allele on the X chromosome. Males have only one X chromosome and cannot, therefore, be heterozygotes for any X-linked trait. The adjective is hemizygous.

Heterogeneity   In genetic terms, the variability or dissimilarity in phenotypes that can be produced by identical alleles. The term is also used to describe similar phenotypes resulting from multiple loci.

Heterozygote   An individual having two different alleles at a given genetic locus, one of which is the normal or wild-type allele. The adjective is heterozygous. Individuals having two different *mutant* alleles at the same genetic locus are usually referred to as double heterozygotes.

Homeostasis   The steady state of individuality in the face of environmental influences, genetic heterogeneity, and developmental phenomena that include growth, differentiation, and maturation. See chapter 2.

Homozygote   An individual having a pair of identical alleles at a given genetic locus. The adjective is homozygous.

Imprinting   The term that describes the differing phenotypes of some genetically determined syndromes depending on the sex of the parent from whom the mutant allele is inherited. See chapter 1.

Incidence   The *rate* of occurrence in a specific population; for example, overall incidence of Down syndrome is approximately one in 650 live births.

Kabuki syndrome   An uncommon autosomal recessive condition first described in Japan and so named because the facies of affected individuals reminded the syndrome's describers of the facial appearance created by the make-up used in the famous Japanese Kabuki theater. The palpebral fissures are remarkably long, usually with eversion of the lateral part of the lower lid, the eyebrows are high arched and often sparse laterally, and there tends to be persistence of the fetal fingerpads (see Figure 3–23). Postnatal growth failure and mental retardation are consistent features.

Linkage   Genes present on the same chromosome are said to be linked if they are transmitted together in meiosis more frequently than expected by chance. The more closely the loci are situated, the more likely they are to segregate together so that the linkage will be detectable. Compare with **synteny**.

Macroglossia   Excessively large tongue seen in the mucopolysaccharidoses (e.g., Hurler's syndrome) and other lysosomal storage diseases, congenital hypothyroidism (cretinism), Beckwith-Wiedemann syndrome, and others (if you enter macroglossia in OMIM on-line, you'll get a list of 18 syndromes!). In Down syndrome, the tongue is protuberant primarily because of hypotonia rather than enlargement.

Mendelian or monogenic inheritance   A trait that is determined entirely or primarily by one gene.

Penetrance   An all-or-none term indicating the frequency of expression of a genotype. If there is no detectable manifestation of the genotype, the trait is said to be nonpenetrant or to show lack of penetrance. If there is even a minor detectable manifestation, the gene is penetrant. This term is often used incorrectly in reference to **expressivity**.

Pharmacogenetics   The study of variability in drug response due to heredity. See **pharmacogenomics**.

Pharmacogenomics   The field of study concerned with development of novel drugs based on newly discovered genes. In practice, the term can be used interchangeably with **pharmacogenetics**.

Phenotype   The observable physical, biochemical, or physiological expression of a gene or group of genes, including the influences of the individual's development from conception to adulthood and the environment to which he or she is exposed.

Philtrum   The groove in the midline of the upper lip; it can be absent, too long, or too short in a variety of syndromes.

Poland's syndrome   Unilateral and highly variable underdevelopment of an upper limb along with aplasia or hypoplasia of the sternal head of the pectoralis major. Other ipsilateral muscle aplasias around the shoulder girdle can occur (serratus anterior, latissimus dorsi) and there can be breast aplasia in females. The occurrence is overwhelmingly sporadic. The accepted cause is an interruption of the early embryonic blood supply involving the subclavian and vertebral arteries and their branches.

Polyploid   Having any multiple of the haploid number of chromosomes other than the normal diploid.

Prader-Willi syndrome   Profound hypotonia is usually the earliest sign, followed by obesity in later childhood, and an almost insatiable appetite. Most patients have a typical round face with almond-shaped eyes, and the hands and feet are small. Intellectual deficits and severe behavioral problems are almost invariable. The cause is a mutation in the long arm of chromosome 15 adjacent to the centromere, usually in the form of a paternally inherited deletion readily detected by FISH analysis (see chapter 1 under "Genomic Imprinting").

Prevalence   The number of cases present in a population at a given time; for example, the number of white school-age children in North America with dyslexia.

Rubinstein-Taybi syndrome   An almost always sporadic condition now known to be due to a microdeletion in the short arm of chromosome 16. It is characterized by microcephaly and a typical face with a prominent beaked nose (see Figure 3–15), a broad fleshy bridge, and often a deviated septum. The eyes are down slanted, often with epicanthal folds, strabismus, or coloboma. The thumbs and great toes are almost always strikingly broad. The paper by Villavicencio, et al (chapter 3, reference 2) presents a fascinating insight into the possible etiology.

Short sternum   Seen in trisomy 18 as part of the general small size of features characterizing that chromosome anomaly.

Smith-Lemli-Opitz syndrome   A highly variable autosomal recessive condition characterized by mental retardation along with multiple congenital anomalies, including growth retardation, facial dysmorphism, syndactyly of toes 2 and 3, postaxial polydactyly, and genital anomalies. It is caused by a defect in cholesterol synthesis with a generalized deficiency of cholesterol and accumulation of its precursors, 7- and 8-dehydrocholesterol. The specific molecular defect lies in the Sonic hedgehog pathway.

Syndrome   A group of reproducible (but often quite variable) manifestations that together are characteristic of a specific disorder or disease; usually but not always each syndrome is due to a common underlying mechanism. An example of the latter: holoprosencephaly syndrome can be inherited as an autosomal recessive trait or result from trisomy 13.

Synteny   The presence of two or more genes on the same chromosome regardless of whether they are close enough together for detection of linkage.

Teeth   Figure 3–17 depicts the typical conical incisors of X-linked ecto-dermal dysplasia along with hypodontia. Other features of the condition include aplasia or hypoplasia of sweat glands with risk of severe high fevers, sparse to absent scalp and body hair, and hypoplastic nipples.

Teratogen   A biological or physical agent that interferes with normal embryonic development and thus can cause congenital anomalies.

Treacher Collins syndrome   An autosomal dominant syndrome charac-terized by abnormal ears, often with hearing loss; micrognathia; midfacial hypoplasia; lower-lid coloboma; and projection of scalp hair onto the lat-eral cheek (see Figure 3–27). Note the absence of a hyphen; it's one man's name!

Uniparental disomy   The presence of two copies of a specific chromo-some, or a portion of a chromosome, inherited from one of the parents with no portion of that chromosome from the other parent.

X inactivation or the Lyon hypothesis   The inactivation in early embryo-genesis of most of the genes on one of the two X chromosomes in each somatic cell of the normal mammalian female in order to achieve dosage compensation. See chapter 1.

Index